ROCKY MOUNTAIN SPOTTED FEVER

ROCKY MOUNTAIN SPOTTED FEVER

By

JERRY K. AIKAWA, M.D.

Associate Professor of Medicine
University of Colorado School of Medicine
Denver, Colorado

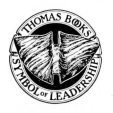

CHARLES C THOMAS • PUBLISHER
Springfield • Illinois • U.S.A.

Published and Distributed Throughout the World by
CHARLES C THOMAS • PUBLISHER
BANNERSTONE HOUSE
301-327 East Lawrence Avenue, Springfield, Illinois, U.S.A.
NATCHEZ PLANTATION HOUSE
735 North Atlantic Boulevard, Fort Lauderdale, Florida, U.S.A.

With THOMAS BOOKS careful attention is given to all details of manufacturing and design. It is the Publisher's desire to present books that are satisfactory as to their physical qualities and artistic possibilities and appropriate for their particular use. THOMAS BOOKS will be true to those laws of quality that assure a good name and good will.

Printed in the United States of America
X-2

TO
C.

Preface

This is the biography of Rocky Mountain spotted fever, a disease which is uniquely all-American: discovered during the westward expansion of the republic; suffered by the pioneers; studied, identified, understood, and finally conquered, in the main, by American scientists. The development of this knowledge mirrors the unprecedented growth of the medical sciences in this society of free men.

Clinical Rocky Mountain spotted fever lived roughly half a century. It is now moribund. Those of us who have witnessed its ravages on unsuspecting victims do not mourn its disappearance; but some look back nostalgically and wish that radioisotopic tools had become available a few years earlier, so that a better understanding of the intriguing pathologic physiology of this disease might have been obtained. The rickettsia responsible for this illness may still be a useful tool in medical research.

This volume is, in a sense, an experiment in medical education. The modern teacher attempts to present, as palatably and concisely as possible, the logical development of a subject or an idea. To the extent that he is successful, his pupils will be able to add facts to this scaffolding so as to fill in the details and perceive the whole. If, in the process, they acquire a few heroes and become imbued with the tradition of service, self-sacrifice, and devotion in medical research, the greater is the teacher's satisfaction.

Acknowledgments

It is a pleasure to acknowledge the assistance of Dr. Henry T. Ricketts in supplying information concerning his father, Dr. Howard Taylor Ricketts, and to thank the Rocky Mountain Research Laboratory at Hamilton, Montana, for lending me its prized scrapbook. Thanks are also due to Mrs. Jacqueline Z. Reardon, who continues to contribute immeasurably to my efforts in research; to Miss Alberta Plym, whose administrative skills afforded me time to write; to Mrs. Junioretta Zimmerman, who typed the many revisions; and to Mrs. Edward W. Jackson, who provided the editorial assistance which makes this volume readable.

J.K.A.

Contents

ROCKY MOUNTAIN SPOTTED FEVER

CHAPTER I

Early History

1.1 The Geology of the Bitter Root Valley

Some 350 million years ago, most of what is now the United States and Canada was the flooded center of a continent hemmed in by mountainous borders (1). The sea receded and several ice ages followed; glaciers covered even the Rocky Mountains. Finally, some twelve thousand years ago, the last glacier melted northward, leaving at latitude 45° to 46°, longitude 114°, a narrow valley approximately ten miles from east to west and fifty miles from north to south. A river (later named the Bitter Root River) flowed through this valley northward until it joined another river (the Hell Gate River).

The mountain ranges on the west and south of this valley are very high and rugged, reaching an altitude of 10,000 feet. Mount Lo Lo, the highest peak, is perpetually capped by snow. The foothills rise suddenly on the west; there once was considerable timber in these regions, and wild animals and ticks abounded. On the east and north, the mountains are of low altitude and the slope of the foothills is gradual; the tick population was considerably smaller on these slopes. The valley itself was formerly the bottom of a huge lake, and its soil was "wonderfully fertile" (2); in some places the subsoil extended down forty feet. Beach marks were prominent on the surrounding mountains, and the rocks were of the type seen in

3

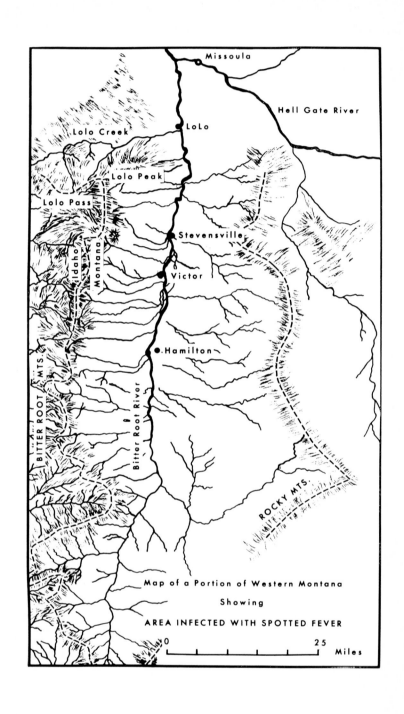

Map of a Portion of Western Montana

Showing

AREA INFECTED WITH SPOTTED FEVER

0   25   Miles

river beds—that is, invariably smooth and round.

Nez Percé and Flat Head tribes of Indians, the sole inhabitants of this region until about 1870, discovered here the "bitter root" plant which covered the landscape each June with its pink blossoms, only to disappear within a few weeks (2). For years, the Indians had used the roots of this plant for medicinal purposes. After grinding the roots to a pulp with a stone mortar and pestle, they rolled them into balls and made them into porridge or tea which was administered for all ailments. The Indians named the river and the valley after this plant.

1.2 Indian Folklore

An old Indian chief told Michie and Parsons (2) that in the spring of the year the Bitter Root Valley was visited by evil spirits, and that it was particularly hazardous at this time to go into certain canyons, as, for instance, Lo Lo Canyon. The precise nature of the danger associated with the evil spirits is not known, and there are no records of serious acute febrile illnesses, suggesting spotted fever, among the Indians in this area.

1.3 The Disease Among Other Indians

That not all Indians were immune and that some occasionally died from spotted fever is indicated in the reports collected by Fricks (3) from Wyoming physicians, who recorded numerous cases, with several deaths, among the Shoshone Indians. Fricks' report mentions that a Mr. Roberts, an Episcopal missionary to the Shoshone and Arapaho Indians for thirty years, had seen probably fifty to seventy-five cases of Rocky Mountain spotted fever,

---

←—⧼   FIGURE 1. Map of the Bitter Root Valley.

with several deaths. The majority of cases occurred between 1890 and 1900 among the Shoshone squaws who went into the mountains to chop wood during early summer. The missionary did not recall any cases among the Arapahos who lived out of the foothills. The Shoshones, unlike the Arapahos, were very much afraid of spotted fever and had a superstition associating the gopher with the disease.

1.4 The White Settlers

History records that after the Bitter Root Valley was evacuated by the Indians and settled by white men (about 1890), a few cases of "black measles," almost all of them fatal, occurred every spring and summer. The early settlers recognized that, as the first warm days of spring arrived, ticks appeared by the millions on the western slopes. They were found on all animals roaming in the fields and also on plants, especially hay. Some of the early settlers had the insight to associate the appearance of ticks with the disease, and so named the disease *tick fever*. Another name given to it was *spotted fever*.

CHAPTER II

Early Clinical Descriptions of Rocky Mountain Spotted Fever

2.1 Idaho Spotted Fever

The first detailed description of spotted fever was published in 1899 by Dr. Edward E. Maxey (4) of Boise City, Idaho. He called attention to the "so-called spotted fever of Idaho" as "an acute, endemic, non-contagious but probably infectious, febrile disease, characterized clinically by a continuous moderately high fever, severe arthritic and muscular pains, and a profuse petechial or purpuric eruption in the skin, appearing first on the ankles, wrists, and forehead, but rapidly spreading to all parts of the body." This type of spotted fever occurred in southern Idaho, on the western side of the Bitter Root Mountains, among sheepherders who worked along the southern foothills of the Boise mountains. The cases seemed to be limited largely to the north side of the Snake River Valley from the settlements of Seven Devils to Haley, and to occur between the latter part of March and the middle of July. The mortality was about 3 per cent.

2.2 Bitter Root Spotted Fever

The first account of the more deadly type of spotted fever characteristic of the Bitter Root Valley was published in July, 1902, by McCullough (5). In his own

7

experience with thirty-six cases seen over a period of twelve years, the mortality was 75 per cent. The cases of spotted fever in the Bitter Root Valley appeared to be more or less confined to valleys, and were seen most often in the foothills on the west side of the river. They occurred only from March through September, and were most numerous in April, May, and June. Both sexes and all ages were subject to the disease, but it was most common in males from twenty-one to forty and in females from eleven to forty. A very large percentage of the patients lived on farms or were connected with the lumbering industry. About 90 per cent gave a history of exposure to wet or cold.

2.3 Geologic Relationship of Idaho and Bitter Root Spotted Fever

Just why cases of spotted fever were so much more numerous and so much less severe in southern Idaho than in the Bitter Root Valley of Montana (the mortality being about 3 per cent in the former and 75 per cent in the latter) has never been explained. Neither is it known in which state the disease first appeared. Geologically, the two infected areas communicate through Lo Lo Canyon, a pass in the Bitter Root Mountains where the most virulent type of the disease occurs. It is probable that the disease spread from one state to the other through this pass.

2.4 Clinical Description

The early clinical descriptions (4-7) of spotted fever were so complete that nothing new has been added to them subsequently. The following description is a composite of these reports.

Seasonal Incidence. Rocky Mountain spotted fever occurs almost wholly in the spring. The first cases usually appear in March after the snow melts, and the incidence reaches its maximum during May and June. Few cases occur during July.

Incubation and Onset. The incubation period seems to range from three to twelve days. The onset is usually accompanied by a chill, although this may be preceded by a few days of malaise with anorexia and chilly sensations. From the beginning of the clinical symptoms the patient has severe general pains referred to the bones and muscles, back and joints. The pains are most severe in the calf muscles, the large joints, and the lumbar region of the back. Headache is common and usually severe. Most patients are ill enough to be bedridden on the second day of symptoms.

The face is flushed and the conjunctivas are injected. Photophobia is usually present, and there may be epistaxis. A very common sign is a hacking cough without production of sputum. The spleen is uniformly enlarged and tender.

Temperature. Before the initial chill, the patient usually has only minimal fever in the evening. After the chill, the temperature rises fairly rapidly, reaching 102° to 104° F on the second day and continuing to rise gradually to a maximum of 104° to 105° F in the second week. The maximum temperature is reached more quickly in the virulent Montana cases than in the Idaho type of the disease. In severe cases of the type seen in the Bitter Root Valley, the temperature reaches 106° to 107° F and may remain this high until death.

The maximum temperature persists during the second week of the disease, with slight morning drops. In patients who recover, the temperature begins to fall by lysis at about the end of the second week, and becomes normal about the end of the third week. For a few days after recovery it may go to 98° F or below. In fatal cases the temperature may drop to normal or subnormal and then rise again eighteen to twenty-four hours before death. Death occurs most commonly between the sixth and twelfth day of the clinical disease (from three to seven days after the eruption appears).

Pulse and Respiration. The pulse is at first full and strong, but it gradually loses volume and strength and increases in rapidity. Both pulse and respiration are disproportionately rapid for the patient's temperature. The pulse ranges from 110 to 140 per minute, and a pulse of 120 with a temperature of 102° F is not uncommon. The respiratory rate is usually thirty to forty per minute. A rapid increase in the pulse and respiratory rates is a bad prognostic sign. The pulse rate may reach 150 per minute a few days before death, and the respiratory rate may rise to sixty in the terminal phase.

Eruption. The rash, which usually appears between the third and the fifth day of fever (most often on the third), shows a remarkable uniformity in its development and its characteristics. It appears first on the wrists, ankles, and back; then on the forehead, arms, legs, and cheeks; finally it is seen on the abdomen, where it is least marked. The efflorescence of the rash takes place over a period of twenty-four to thirty-six hours, although after this the palms, soles, scalp, and mucous membranes of the cheek, palate, pharynx, and fauces may become sites for the eruption. With the development of the rash the general aches and pains ameliorate, but the fever continues.

The rash first consists of rose-colored macules, varying in diameter from less than 1 mm to 5 mm. These are not elevated, and disappear upon pressure. The spots soon become deep red or purplish and increase in size; they often become confluent, thus giving the skin a diffuse, marbled appearance. After they have been present for several days (between the sixth and the tenth days of the disease), the spots no longer disappear upon pressure and the rash becomes distinctly petechial in character. In severe cases large areas of cutaneous and subcutaneous hemorrhage develop. Frequently the skin assumes a glazed appearance in the second week, and the thighs may show a peculiar dusky reddish or bluish mottling.

The rash begins to disappear with the subsidence of fever, but the sites of the petechiae remain as pigmented spots. These may persist for weeks or months, becoming demonstrable when the skin is chilled, or after strenuous exercise or a hot bath. In severe cases, the skin of certain dependent parts frequently becomes necrotic in the third week of the disease. This necrosis is most common in the scrotum, prepuce, fingers, toes, and lobes of the ears. Necrosis may also affect the soft palate. Desquamation follows recovery, and extends over the whole body. In exceptional cases casts may be formed over the sites of large hemorrhages on the palms and soles.

Nervous System. Restlessness and insomnia are common throughout the illness and are among its most distressing symptoms. Hyperesthesia is frequent and may be severe; the slightest touch, movement of the bed, or even the weight of the bedclothes may cause extreme pain.

In severe cases the patient usually becomes delirious during the height of the fever, and in fatal cases coma most often precedes death by a few hours to a day.

Gastrointestinal Symptoms. Constipation is present from the onset and persists throughout the disease. Icterus appears in the second week of the disease, but is never very marked. Vomiting may occur during the onset and again later, preceding a fatal outcome. Massive gastrointestinal bleeding sometimes develops before death.

Urine. The volume is decreased and albumin may appear in small amounts. In general, the urinary findings are those common to severe fevers in which there is no special renal involvement.

Blood. There is slight leukocytosis, with counts ranging up to 12,000. The large mononuclear leukocytes, except for the large lymphocytes, show a striking increase in number. The eosinophils are decreased in number, and may be entirely absent.

The red cell count decreases as the disease progresses, and may fall below 3,500,000 per cubic millimeter before death. The coagulation time is increased.

Complications. Pneumonia is the one complication, and it is infrequent.

2.5 Treatment

At the time these early clinical descriptions were written, there was no specific treatment. Cold baths were recommended, although antipyretics were considered undesirable. Morphine and hyoscine were recommended for allaying symptoms related to the central nervous system. "In general, the therapeutic measures should be directed towards conserving the strength of the patient and allaying discomfort, thus insuring the most favorable circumstances for the natural forces of the body against the infection" (6).

The following drugs had been found to have no beneficial action: quinine, coal-tar products, calcium sulfide, creosote, various forms of arsenic, and injections of sodium citrate.

CHAPTER III

Early Investigations on Spotted Fever

3.1 The Beginning

The organized battle against spotted fever may be said to have begun in March, 1901, when the Montana State Board of Health was created (8). Early in April of that year, the governor of the state received an urgent appeal from the people of the Bitter Root Valley to do something about spotted fever, a mysterious disease which had appeared every spring for about ten years, killing a score of victims. It attacked only those who had been up in the mountains west of the Bitter Root River. The local residents said that it had something to do with drinking melted snow, which was about all a shepherd or stockman could find to drink when he went into the foothills with his animals in the spring.

3.2 The Work of Wilson and Chowning

The problem was turned over to Dr. A. F. Longeway, the first secretary of the Montana State Board of Health, who asked for help from the Board of Health of Minnesota. So it was that on May 2, 1902, Dr. Louis B. Wilson, a young pathologist who was later to become head of the Mayo Foundation, arrived in Missoula from Minneapolis to start research on spotted fever. During his first ten days in Missoula, he saw three patients with spotted fever. All died, and he was present at each autopsy. On May 26 a second pathologist, Dr. W. M. Chowning, arrived from Minneapolis to assist Wilson. In a little over a month, the two investigators saw a total of seven persons succumb to the fever.

After two seasons of work, Wilson and Chowning had obtained records of 126 cases of spotted fever (in which the mortality was 87 per cent), and had made the first postmortem examinations and the first studies of the blood during life (9). They reported finding a supposed intracorpuscular protozoan parasite, a *Piroplasma*, which was thought to be similar to that known to cause Texas fever, a disease of cattle which is transmitted by ticks. This part of their work did not prove valid, and their findings are still unexplained.

On the basis of their studies, Wilson and Chowning wrote an account of the clinical and anatomic phases of Rocky Mountain spotted fever (9). This report, while containing some erroneous conclusions regarding etiology, nevertheless contributed many valuable facts, particularly as to pathology and epidemiology.

Wilson and Chowning were eager to return to Montana the next season to continue their studies, but the Montana Board of Health did not have the funds to pay them.

3.3 The Tick Theory

Probably the first physician in Montana to suspect the role of ticks in spotted fever was Dr. Earle Strain, a physician practicing in Great Falls, Montana, who was a good friend of Dr. A. F. Longeway. Dr. Longeway told Wilson about Strain's theory. Noting that every one of the seven persons who died had been bitten by a tick,

Wilson and Chowning agreed that there appeared to be a causal relationship. Their report (9) contains their conclusion that the disease was transmitted by the wood tick of the locality. They suggested that the Columbian ground squirrel (gopher) might be the source of infection for the ticks.

The tick transmission theory aroused considerable local opposition in Montana, partly from physicians who occasionally found no evidence of tick bites in their cases, but chiefly from those interested in the economic development of the infested localities.

3.4 First Federal Participation

Federal participation in the study of Rocky Mountain spotted fever began in 1903, when Passed Assistant Surgeon John F. Anderson, of the Public Health and Marine Hospital Service, was assigned to Montana to investigate the disease. Anderson (6) confirmed Wilson's and Chowning's finding of *Piroplasma* in the blood of patients, and supported the theory of tick transmission.

3.5 The Stiles Report

Early in 1904, C. W. Stiles, Chief of the Division of Zoology, Hygienic Laboratory, United States Public Health and Marine Hospital Service, was detailed to study the disease from a zoological point of view. Anderson had previously sent the Montana ticks back to Stiles in Washington. Stiles found that they belonged to the genus *Dermacentor,* and named them *Dermacentor andersoni.* (This is the same tick that Banks had named *Dermacentor venustus.*)

The report which Stiles submitted (7) contained the most complete summary of knowledge of this disease that had been written up to that time. Stiles noted that in 200 hours of microscopic study he was unable to find a *Piroplasma* in fresh blood from nine patients with spotted fever or in stained blood from these and several additional cases. Moreover, he wrote, "Chowning was unable to demonstrate the parasite to us in the fresh and stained blood of a typical case . . . Indications are not lacking that at least some of the stages of the supposed *Piroplasma hominis* consist in reality of vacuoles, blood platelets, blood dust, artifacts, and tertian malaria parasites." Stiles also flatly contradicted the tick theory.

3.6 Direct Transmission of Spotted Fever from Man to Man

Remarkable transmission experiments with ticks on man were made in 1905 by L. P. McCalla of Boise, Idaho, but were not published until 1908 (10). McCalla removed a tick from a patient with spotted fever and, with the consent of the subjects, allowed it to feed for forty-eight hours upon the arm of a man (a healthy jail prisoner) and, immediately after removal, upon the leg of a woman, where it remained attached for ten to twenty-four hours. After an incubation period of nine days, the man had a typical case of spotted fever of medium severity, with fever lasting eight or nine days. Spotted fever also appeared in the woman after an incubation period of three days. She had fever up to 101° F, lasting four or five days and accompanied by a rash which was regarded as typical of a mild case. These experiments, unknown to Ricketts and antedating his transmission experiments, are the only recorded instances in which spotted fever was transmitted by a tick from man to man.

CHAPTER IV

Contributions of
Howard T. Ricketts

Refutation of the tick theory by Stiles and his failure to confirm Wilson's and Chowning's findings left the etiology of spotted fever still in doubt.

Unexpected help appeared in 1906 in the person of Dr. Howard Taylor Ricketts, who came to Montana from the University of Chicago of his own accord. Because the experts disagreed, he considered it an opportune time for the *Piroplasma* theory to be proved or disproved by a third person without prejudice for or against it.

4.1 Arrival in Missoula

"I arrived in Missoula, Montana, April 21, 1906, equipped for the bacteriologic and hematologic study of the so-called Rocky Mountain spotted fever and for the study of the infectious agent by means of animal inoculations" (11). So begins Ricketts' series of communications on spotted fever. Those who observed him noted that he brought the finest equipment available and employed the most careful technique. "Unlike his predecessors, he was not content to make sporadic buggy trips into the tick infested regions, but went for days at a time into the canyons toward the mountains; and stayed in Stevensville to confer with local doctors" (8).

4.2 Inability to Confirm Reports of Wilson and Chowning

Ricketts initially attempted to confirm the findings of Wilson and Chowning, but he was unsuccessful in identifying a parasite in human blood or in culturing the organism in bacteriologic media.

TABLE I

CHRONOLOGY OF THE STUDIES OF HOWARD T. RICKETTS
IN MONTANA DURING THE SEASON OF 1906 (11)

April 21 Arrived in Missoula, Montana. Pitched tent on lawn of Great Northern Hospital and started work.

April 27 Injected defibrinated blood from spotted fever patient into two rabbits intravenously. Negative results.

May 5 Injected two guinea pigs intraperitoneally with blood from patient with spotted fever. In both, fever and scrotal and testicular swelling developed. One died on the eleventh day. Second group of guinea pigs injected with blood from these two animals; a clinical illness developed in one. *Actual transference of infection established.*

May 6 Repeated rabbit experiment. Experiment considered not satisfactory, but the animal did become ill, with fever as high as 104.8° F.

May 20 a) Inoculated two guinea pigs with blood from another patient with spotted fever. Death at seven and eight days. Unable to perpetuate infection past second passage by direct transference.
b) Injected one monkey with blood from a human case of spotted fever. The febrile disease that followed was characterized by the cyanotic face and injected conjunctivas typical of spotted fever in man.

June 11 a) Studied filterability of the "virus." Filtered serum had no discoverable effect on animals.
b) Injected second monkey with blood from a human case. The animal died on the ninth day of an illness characterized by erythema of the perineum. Illness in second-passage monkey characterized by fever (to 106.7° F), perineal redness, and hemorrhagic eruptions on scrotum, buttocks, legs, and back.

June 19 Attached a small female tick to an infected guinea pig.

June 23 Attached the same tick to a normal guinea pig, in which a febrile illness developed.

June 11-
Sept. 6   Alternated the infection between monkeys and guinea pigs,
            and preserved the "virus" in experimental animals.
Oct.
through
Nov.   Succeeded in perpetuating the infection in guinea pigs.
May
through
Aug.   Studied the life cycle of the tick under laboratory conditions.

4.3 Successful Transmission of Infection in Guinea Pigs

The remarkable rapidity and unerring logic with which
Ricketts attacked the problem are evident in the chronology of his accomplishments during the first season
that he worked with spotted fever (Table I). Initially
he tried to transmit the infection to rabbits by the
intravenous injection of defibrinated blood from a patient
with spotted fever. Since the rabbits remained well, he
next tried another species of experimental animal—the
guinea pig. "Astonishing and strikingly positive results
were obtained" immediately (11). In two male guinea
pigs which were given intraperitoneal injections of blood
from a human case of spotted fever, the development of
a febrile illness was followed by swelling of the testicles
and scrotum, and hemorrhages into the skin of the
scrotum. Ricketts was able to effect subsequent passages
of the infection in guinea pigs by inoculating them with
heart blood and splenic emulsions from the original two
guinea pigs.

4.4 Filterability of the "Virus"

To determine the filterability of the "virus" and its

FIGURE 2. Ricketts' laboratory and sleeping quarters in Missoula,
            Montana, 1906 and 1907.   ⟫⟶

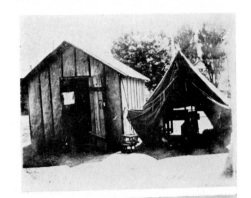

1906

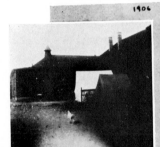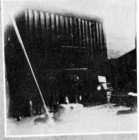

1907

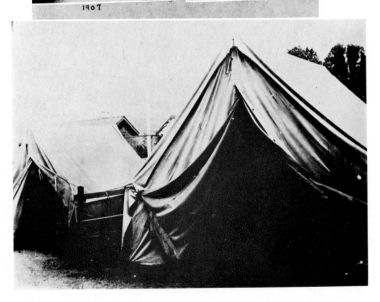

distribution among the constitutents of blood, Ricketts
inoculated guinea pigs with fresh defibrinated blood,
washed corpuscles, and unfiltered serum from patients
with spotted fever. A typical and fatal infection was
produced in each case, whereas serum filtered through a
small Berkefeld filter under low pressure had no discoverable effect. Ricketts concluded that "the condition
produced in the guinea pig is an infection and not an
intoxication" (12).

4.5 Infection of a Monkey

Defibrinated blood from a patient with spotted fever
was then injected intravenously into a healthy and fairly
large Rhesus monkey, which became ill on the second day.
Fever (ranging from 103.1° to 105.3° F) continued until
the tenth day and then subsided. The monkey's face was
cyanotic and the conjunctivas were injected—characteristic
signs of spotted fever in man. Ricketts was then hopeful
of adapting the "virus" to guinea pigs in an effort to
produce a vaccine.

4.6 Transmission by the Wood Tick

Having successfully transmitted Rocky Mountain spotted fever to the guinea pig and monkey, Ricketts next
tested the theory of transmission by the wood tick (12). A
small female tick was placed at the base of the ear of a
guinea pig inoculated intraperitoneally eight days previously with blood from a patient who had died of spotted
fever. After being allowed to feed for two days, the tick

FIGURE 3. Notes from Ricketts' notebook concerning the first
successful inoculation of a guinea pig with blood from a patient
with spotted fever.   ⫸—→

Table I

B.P. 1.   Maggie Cortsen,   5/5/06   †

Guinea-pig inoculations.
Blood taken the 6th day of the disease,

I ☞ Blood drawn at 1 P.m. and defibrinated at once. Inoculations made at 7.30
P.m., hence blood was 6½ hrs. old, and
was kept at out-door temperature,

I. Fuchs in our nose. About 500 grams,
3 c.c. defib. blood into peritoneal cavity.
Temp. before injection. 102 ,
                                102.3   a.m.   5/1
    [2 controls,   102.
                               102.3]

Skipped several days, being in Butte.
5/12/06. — 6 days. — Emaciated — Temp. 104.8
(nor. 5.p 102.3 and 102.6), Scrotum
swollen and ecchymotic. Testes somewhat
tender.
5/13/06 — a.m. temp. 103.8°. Swelling of
scrotum more marked as are hemorrhages.
No hemorrhages on skin elsewhere. No gross
lesions of genitalia are found. Weakness and
emaciation are greatly increased.
Skin over scrotum incised superficially, and
a sero-sanguinolent fluid escapes. This, stained
with Löfflers and Harris' stains as well as
when examined fresh shows many groups of
cocci -(staph.) some in pairs and others
in chains of 4 to 6. Slides saved.
Blood smears from blood of ear stained with
Nasticys and Harris. Nothing found on super-
ficial examination.
5/15/06 - died at about 10 P.m. Sick 7 days.
Body greatly emaciated. Condition of skin of scrotum previously noted. No other hemorrhagic
                    (over)

was removed and then attached, two days later, to the base of the ear of a normal female guinea pig. After three and one half days, the latter animal began to have fever, ranging up to 106.4° F; the external genitalia became swollen and congested. The fever left after seven days, and the animal recovered. Because he had no more guinea pigs, Ricketts was unable to transmit the infection further at that time.

It should be stressed that adequate controls were used in this experiment: uninfected ticks were allowed to feed on normal guinea pigs, which did not show a rise in temperature; and guinea pigs were kept for two weeks in the box occupied by the infected animals. The fact that these animals also failed to show any abnormal temperature argued against transmission of the infection by mere association with the excretions of infected animals. "The knowledge so far gained may well be taken into account in instituting prophylactic measures against the disease" (12).

4.7 Tissue Distribution; Active Immunity

Ricketts was unable at first to perpetuate the infection in guinea pigs alone and was forced to alternate inoculations between monkeys and guinea pigs (13). He subsequently found that the infection could be perpetuated in guinea pigs alone by inoculating them with blood or organs taken from infected guinea pigs between the third and fifth days of fever (14). He next studied the distribution of the virus in the body of the infected animal and found that the lymph nodes, spleen, bone marrow, testicles, liver, kidney, and brain were all infective (13, 14). The disease could be transmitted from one animal to another by the bite of either the male or the female tick (14). Ricketts demonstrated that one attack in a monkey conferred active immunity and concluded that man probably acquires a similar immunity (13). Some of the experimental results suggested to Ricketts that "toxic substances" are liberated into the blood during the infection.

4.8 Life Cycle of the Tick

During this period Ricketts was also studying, under laboratory conditions, the life history of the tick which was the suspected carrier of the disease. (Ricketts called the tick he worked with *Dermacentor occidentalis.* Later investigation proved this classification wrong, the tick being the same one now known as *Dermacentor andersoni.*) He found that this tick passes through a larval stage and subsequently molts twice before reaching the adult form, the cycle from egg to adult requiring about three months under laboratory conditions. The tick leaves the host in order to molt (13).

4.9 Subsequent Studies in Chicago

In the latter part of September, 1906, Ricketts returned to Chicago, where he continued studies on the distribution of the virus in the body fluids; its viability and resistance under different conditions; its filterability and certain other properties; and the preservation of the virus by uninterrupted passage through guinea pigs.

4.10 Transmission of the Virus in Ticks

Ricketts came back to the Bitter Root Valley for a second season of work in 1907. By the end of that year, he was able to report that the adult male and female and the nymph of the Rocky Mountain wood tick are able to acquire and transmit spotted fever (14). The larva may acquire the disease and remain infective during the nymphal stage. The virus may be transmitted from an infected female to her young through the eggs. The virus exits in both the gut and the salivary glands of the infected tick (15), but is not highly destructive for the tick.

> At least two important steps may now be taken in an aggressive fight against the disease: first, a thorough dissemination of the knowledge that the tick is the agent of infection; second, a massive reduction of the number of ticks in infected districts. . . . It is known locally that the number of ticks in the Bitter Root Valley has increased enormously as greater numbers of domesticated animals have been introduced, and the latter now seems to be the chief host for the tick (14).

4.11 Winter Visit to the Bitter Root Valley

In December, 1907, Ricketts again visited the Bitter Root Valley in order to determine the exact form in which the tick survives the winter, and under what conditions. He found that infected ticks occur in nature and that small wild animals such as squirrels are the source of the virus (15). Ricketts concluded that spotted fever in man depends simply on the accidental bite of an adult tick carrying an active virus. The peculiar seasonal prevalence is explained by the facts that only adult ticks find their way to man and that they occur only in the spring.

4.12 The Third Season of Study

In February, 1908, Ricketts suggested the development of a serum for the prevention of Rocky Mountain spotted fever. He already had an immune serum obtained from a horse which, if injected into experimental animals within three days of the tick bite, thoroughly protected the recipient (16). "Successful vaccination, not hitherto reported, has been accomplished by the injection of the tissues and eggs of virulent ticks (rich in bacilli) after the material has been sterilized either by desiccation or by chloroform" (17, 18). He outlined for the Montana Board of Health the first definitive program for the control of the disease: a plan to cut down the tick population of the Bitter Root valley by preventing the female ticks from reaching maturity on cattle and horses. He suggested that livestock be treated with oil and carding and that the ground squirrels be exterminated.

4.13 First Microscopic Description of a Causative Microorganism

In 1909, Ricketts demonstrated a parasitic microorganism in the blood of human beings, guinea pigs, and monkeys which he thought bore a specific relationship to Rocky Mountain spotted fever (19). By Giemsa staining, he found two minute "somewhat lanceolate chromatin-staining bodies, separated by a slight amount of eosin-staining substance." He thought he saw similar organisms in the tissues and eggs of infected ticks. These small organisms were agglutinated, under proper circumstances, by blood from an immune guinea pig. Because he was unable to cultivate the microorganism, however, Ricketts was unwilling to claim yet that this was the specific organism causing Rocky Mountain spotted fever.

4.14 Legislative Appropriation to Continue Ricketts' Studies (8)

The health authorities of Montana were so favorably impressed with Ricketts's studies that the 1909 legislature

appropriated $6,000 for Ricketts' use alone, in order to
ensure his return for the next two seasons and the continuation of his studies on Rocky Mountain spotted fever.
The Montana Board of Examiners, however, was not
research-minded. When it found that the 1909 legislature
had appropriated more money than the state treasury
contained, the spotted fever research was deleted and
Ricketts was informed that the money was not available.
In spite of this news, he waited from April until July for
release of the funds before finally accepting an invitation
from Mexico to study typhus fever. He hoped that this
study would throw light on spotted fever, since there is
considerable similarity between the two diseases. In
December, 1909, the Board of Examiners finally released
the $6,000 appropriation for Ricketts, but it was then
too late.

4.15 Death of Ricketts

The delay of nine months in releasing the appropria-
tion of $6,000 may have changed the course of medical
science, since it led to Ricketts' trip to Mexico and his
death. Ricketts wrote the Montana Board of Health that
he could not abandon the work which he had well under
way in Mexico City, but would try to be in Montana on
May 1, 1910. Ricketts was not able to keep his word:
he died of typhus fever on May 3, 1910.

4.16 Biography of Ricketts

The name of Howard T. Ricketts was appropriately
perpetuated in science by da Rocha-Lima when, in 1916,
he gave the name *Rickettsia* to the group of microbes
Ricketts had discovered. What manner of man was this
who, in such a short period of time and often working

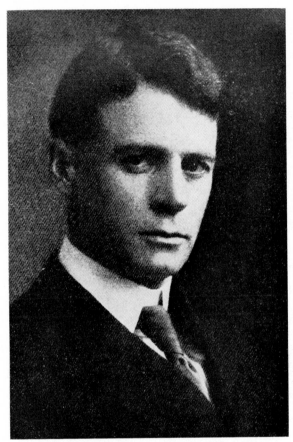

FIGURE 4. Howard T. Ricketts, 1871-1910.

under crude conditions, brought facts to light with such brilliance and accuracy that he laid the foundations for most of the major approaches subsequently used by others in the study of the rickettsial diseases?

Howard Taylor Ricketts was born on a farm in Hancock County near the town of Findlay in northwestern Ohio, February 9, 1871. His father, Andrew Duncan Ricketts, and his mother, Nancy Jane, were both natives of Ohio. His father had been a soldier in the Civil War. Howard was the second son in a family of five brothers and two sisters. When he was seven, his family moved to Champaign County, Ohio, near the village of Fisher, where his father was engaged in the grain business. Here Howard spent the next ten years of his life.

The nearby Eagle Creek offered ample opportunities for fishing, swimming, boating, and hunting. Although hunting was Howard's greatest delight, he was also fond of music and learned to play the piano well enough to accompany his own singing. He was popular with his playmates and was considered a "regular boy."

Of his happy boyhood days he later wrote:

> When I was a boy, I used to ride a horse a good deal and, above everything else, I loved, in summer, when the rain was warm, to ride against the wind with the rain beating in my face. I used to drive all the neighbors' cows to the pasture, a mile and a half away, for a certain amount each month. I usually rode bare-back and it was then I used to love to ride when it was raining, thundering and lightning. I spent many happy days in that little town (20).

There was no high school in this prairie village of five to six hundred people. Howard's parents belonged to that comparatively small number who desired to give their children a college education. They were also religious people and, being Methodists, decided to send Howard to Northwestern University at Evanston, Illinois. The boy himself had become a member of the Methodist Church, and he welcomed the plan. Entering the academy of the university in 1887, Howard finished his preparation for college in three years. These years expanded his horizon; he relished the association with scholars and the discovery of knowledge in books, and of life itself.

The important event of Howard's second year in the academy was that Miss Myra E. Tubbs of Kirkwood, Illinois, became a member of his class. The acquaintance begun between these two young people at that time was to culminate twelve years later in their marriage. They graduated from the academy together and entered Northwestern at the same time in 1890.

During his sophomore year, at the age of twenty-one, Ricketts decided to follow medicine as a profession. The family physician in his home town had urged him to enter medicine and Miss Myra Tubbs concurred.

Because Howard's parents were intent on giving all their children a college education, they decided to move to a university town so that the children could go through college without leaving home. Partly because Mr. Ricketts' father, brother, and sister resided in Lincoln, Nebraska, where the state university was located, they moved there in 1892. Howard had just finished his sophomore year at Northwestern. He had become very much attached to the university and to the girl who later became his wife (though as yet he had no assurance that the attachment was mutual). Leaving Evanston reluctantly in June, 1892, he returned to Fisher to assist in his family's move.

When he entered the University of Nebraska in the fall as a junior, he took all the scientific courses he could. Then and always he was a faithful and ambitious student. His German professor once said, in addressing the Lincoln alumni, "I tell you Ricketts is a great fellow. Whenever I want to fix my mind on a good example of a student, I think of Ricketts" (20).

Ricketts thoroughly enjoyed university life. He not only possessed unusual ability as a student; he was also a delightful companion and was often seen at parties of young people. He was a member of the glee club and the football squad, and was an enthusiastic amateur photographer. Because of his interest in medicine, he was taken into the office of Dr. Giffen, a prominent physician in Lincoln.

Until the end of his college career Howard had never had to work for his own support, for his father had always provided for him liberally. The financial panic of 1893 changed this situation. Corn sold for as little as six cents a bushel, and Howard's father suffered with the others. During the summer of 1894, he wrote that, in order to provide for the expenses of his medical course, he would "play a triple role for the rest of the summer as newspaper man, paid singer in a church, and as instructor in zoology. My newspaper work occupies my time from four to seven A.M. I have to rustle out pretty early to count the papers and get the boys started on their routes" (20).

In the fall of 1894, young Ricketts began a three-year course of study at the medical school of Northwestern University, in Chicago. For the first time he was dependent upon his own efforts for money to meet his expenses, and he had a desperate struggle. The fall of 1894 was highlighted by his engagement to Myra E. Tubbs, with whom he had been in constant correspondence during the two years that he had been in Lincoln. In spite of his financial difficulties, Howard's first year in medical school passed pleasantly and successfully. He prepared the skeleton of a dog in competition for a prize and won. On Sundays he taught a class in a mission school, a task which he continued through the ensuing summer.

As the college year closed, Ricketts arranged to live with a member of the faculty, Dr. W. H. Allport, who provided him with a room and two meals a day in return for half-time service. His service consisted of attention to the college museum, the study of comparative anatomy, and the preparation of specimens. The summer was a very profitable one to Ricketts. Dr. Allport later wrote of him:

> I never knew a man who was so scientifically trust-worthy and untiring. He never cared about sleep and his soul cried out always for knowledge, knowledge, and more knowledge, and was always unappeased. . . . He was the most persistent and accomplished notetaker I ever came across in my experience as a teacher. He had hundreds and hundreds of notebooks. . . . In every way his life was frank, honest, rich in the pleasure of intellectual achievement and bare of everything which appealed to the luxurious instincts of the lower senses; he was a Spartan, a Flagellant, a Puritan with himself, and, although I never heard him criticize anyone else, the standard which he set for himself in his own life was nothing short of moral and spiritual perfection (20).

Of his own philosophy Howard Ricketts wrote: "I think a busy life and a clear conscience are the two most important factors for one's happiness . . . I think charity is almost the greatest thing in the world and God grant we may all have more of it—charity in our relations to others and strict exactions from our own selves" (20).

Toward the end of his second year Ricketts was promised the position of demonstrator in histology for the next year. He ranked third in a large class, his average for the year being above ninety-six. He was in dire need of financial support; his own resources were exhausted and his father was unable to help at all. That summer he got a room with Dr. T. J. Watkins, paying for it in service.

For some time he prepared his own breakfast and dinner. He earned $25 weekly nursing a patient through the heat of summer, and every $25 meant a month of school the next year. During the latter part of the summer he accompanied Octave Chanute, a pioneer of aviation, on a trip to the dunes, serving as his medical attendant and cook.

Three weeks before the autumn term was to start, Ricketts' resources totaled only about $200, and he had to borrow $100 to pay his tuition. To make matters worse, he discovered that the moths had been busy on his dress suit and cutaway coat. Ricketts wrote: "I used to think it would be very humiliating to be poor, but I don't find it so. I have as much personal pride as ever" (20).

During the winter of 1896 Ricketts' work load proved too heavy, and he had a nervous breakdown. In January, 1897, his friend, the dean of the Northwestern University Medical School, advised him to take six weeks' leave of absence. Although he had cherished an opportunity to take the examinations for intern at the Cook County Hospital, Ricketts gave up hope when he was forced to leave school in the middle of his final year. Fortunately, in spite of his illness and long absence, he was given the appointment, which was to begin in December of 1897.

Ricketts spent the interval between his graduation from medical school and the beginning of his internship in nursing patients, serving as cashier at an amusement park, and acting as locum tenens for a physician in a small community near Chicago. Looking back on the years between college and his internship, he said later, "I have done about everything except to push a banana cart" (20).

Young Dr. Ricketts started his internship at the Cook County Hospital on December 1, 1897. Before long, his

superior scholarship, clearheadedness, and keenness came
to the attention of the staff. Eighteen months of working
with Billings, Herrick, Murphy, and others afforded him
priceless experience, and he worked to the limit of his
strength. His period as intern ended June 1, 1899.

Ricketts' exceptional record at Cook County Hospital
had attracted the attention of the faculty of Rush Medical
College. Dr. J. Nevins Hyde, professor of dermatology at
Rush, offered him a fellowship in skin pathology, a post
established especially for Ricketts at a stipend of $800.
Acceptance of this position gave Ricketts his first opportunity for independent research, and he promptly became
interested in blastomycosis. He continued as a fellow and
assistant at Rush for two years. During this period he
was married to Miss Myra E. Tubbs. He was then twenty-
nine years old. Their marriage had been deferred for six
years, at the strong insistence of a lady who understood
her fiance's increasing desire to make the best preparation
for his life's work.

Ricketts had finally decided on research and teaching
in the field of pathology as that work. His studies on
blastomycosis made him desire to work in the famous
schools and laboratories of Europe. On May 1, 1900,
Dr. and Mrs. Ricketts went abroad. After touring England,
Scotland, and Ireland, they spent three months in Berlin,
where their son Henry—the now eminent Henry T.
Ricketts, M.D., of the University of Chicago—was born.
Their next stop was Vienna, where Ricketts heard from
his old friend and teacher, Dr. Ludvig Hektoen, head of
the department of pathology and bacteriology in the
University of Chicago. Hektoen offered Ricketts a position
in his department, but asked that he first spend several
months working at the Pasteur Institute.

Ricketts' appointment as an associate in pathology at the University of Chicago began on July 1, 1902; his salary was $1,000 per year. He was then thirty-one years of age, but looked young enough to be mistaken for one of his students. At the end of the first year he was promoted to the rank of instructor, with an increase in salary. He continued laboratory studies on blastomycosis, which eventually led to the publication of his book, *Infection, Immunity and Serum Therapy,* in 1906.

Having read about Rocky Mountain spotted fever, Howard Ricketts decided in 1906 to investigate the subject. Financial assistance was secured from the American Medical Association, Missoula and Ravalli counties in Montana, and other sources. The contributions made by this genius during the four years that he worked on spotted fever have already been recounted.

Early in 1910 Ricketts accepted the chair of pathology at the University of Pennsylvania—a position he was never to occupy. When, in the spring of 1909, it appeared that funds would not be available for Ricketts to continue his studies on spotted fever in Montana, he accepted an invitation from the Mexican government to study typhus fever in Mexico City. He and Russell Wilder, his volunteer assistant, began work in Mexico City in December, 1909. They promptly showed that Mexican typhus differed from Rocky Mountain spotted fever in causation and insect transmission. In April, 1910, their discovery of a distinctive microbe in lice and in the blood of typhus patients was announced. On May 3, 1910, Howard Taylor Ricketts died of typhus fever in Mexico City, at the age of forty.

Dr. Ludvig Hektoen, at a memorial service held at the University of Chicago on May 5, 1910, described his former colleague as follows:

Dr. Ricketts was a modest and unassuming man, of great determination and of the highest character, loyal and generous, earnest and genuine in all his doings—a personality of unusual and winning charm. His associates of the hospital and fellowship days, who knew him well, knew his ability and energy, his distinct fondness for the day's work; all looked to him for the more than ordinary achievement. . . . He had early become possessed of noble ideals and had a pure love for the search after truth in his chosen field, which abided with him and gave him a high conception of all his duties and relations and placed a special stamp on his work.

Thus a young and noble career of great achievement and of large service to humanity came to a sudden and heroic end, and a new name was placed on the martyr role of science.

Those near to him knew that he fully understood the danger to which he would be exposed and the risks he would run. He decided he would take these risks, meet the dangers with all possible means of prevention, and do the work that would come to his hands. And so he made the great sacrifice and gave all that a man can give for his fellow-men (23).

A signal honor was shown Dr. Ricketts' memory when President Diaz of Mexico directed that the professors and students of the National Medical School be present when his body was put on the train to Chicago, and that the medical school and Institute of Bacteriology be draped in mourning for three days. Two laboratories carry Ricketts' name: one in Mexico City, the other at the University of Chicago, where a Ricketts prize has also been established. Another tribute was paid to him by the Chicago Pathological Society, whose members contributed voluntarily to the cost of publishing, on the first anniversary of his death, a volume of his contributions to medical science (23).

Of interest are editorials from newspapers of that day. Commented the *Brooklyn Eagle*: "We may thus add one more name to the list of modern martyrs of science who get but a passing thought from the preoccupied people of the United States." The *Chicago Evening Post*, in an editorial written on April 30, before his death, said that Dr. Ricketts "belongs to the small corps of American physicians and scientists who are achieving distinction for their scientific research in the origin and cause of disease."

In an editorial entitled "On the Firing Line," the *Chicago Tribune* for May 6 paid him the following tribute:

> The death of Dr. Howard T. Ricketts adds another name to the long honor roll of science. The endless warfare that mankind has fought against ignorance and its child, disease, has claimed another victim, but the fight goes on. Dr. Ricketts left his unfinished investigations to his fellow workers in the field of medical research. But he left something much more precious to his fellow men—the example of a high courage and devotion in the cause of humanity. Dr. Ricketts died on the firing line of human progress, and it is inspiring to believe, as we may, that he did not die in vain. Mankind is richer for his living and nobler for his dying.

CHAPTER V

Control of the Disease
In the Bitter Root Valley

It could well be that Ricketts' untimely death delayed by several years the control of Rocky Mountain spotted fever in the Bitter Root Valley. Yet, even as those who appreciated Ricketts' genius mourned his loss, other scientists took up the task of understanding and controlling this disease.

5.1 The Entomologists, Willard King and Clarence Birdseye

The scene now shifts to the work of two young entomologists. In 1909 Willard King, who had just finished his junior year at Montana State College, was appointed "agent and expert of the U.S. Bureau of Entomology" to make a tick survey over the Northwestern states. Collaborating with King was Clarence Birdseye, then a student at Amherst College, who was more interested in practical research than in a college degree. (Birdseye later developed frozen foods.) He served as field naturalist for the U.S. Biological Survey. These two discovered that tick larvae and nymphs live on small rodents, while the adult ticks live chiefly on large animals: cattle, horses, mountain goats, elk, and bear (25). Of importance was the finding that the woodchuck, in contrast, harbors both nymphs and full-grown adult ticks.

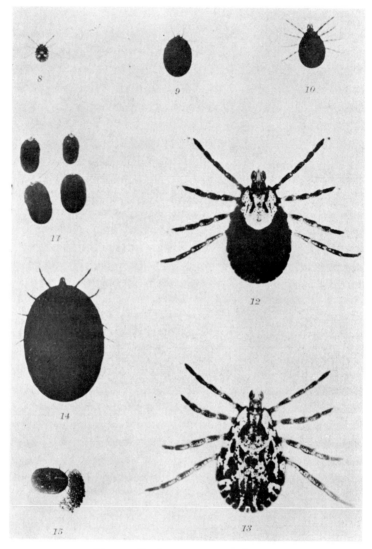

FIGURE 5. *Dermacentor andersoni.*
8. Unfed larva, 8 diameters.
9. Engorged larva, 8 diameters.

5.2 The Tick Cycle

King (26) found that the adult female tick deposits on the ground several thousand eggs, which hatch into six-legged larvae or "seed" ticks. These larvae climb up nearby vegetation and there await the passing of small mammals such as squirrels or mice, to which they attach themselves. After a few days, when fully fed, they drop to the ground and seek a suitably protected place for the molting period. When molting is complete, they emerge as second-stage ticks, or eight-legged nymphs. The nymph may or may not find a host to feed upon the first summer. If not, it secretes itself in a hiding place and hibernates until the next spring, when it comes out ready to feed. The nymphs feed on the same species of small rodents as do the larvae. After about a week of feeding they drop off, hide away for several weeks, then emerge as adult ticks. These also may or may not feed the same summer.

The adult insects follow the same general procedure as the larvae and nymphs. They climb up some weed or grass stalk and, grasping this support with two legs, extend the other six in readiness to cling to the first passing victim, man or animal. Once attached, both male and female ticks feed to repletion, and fertilization takes place on the host animal. Before the resultant death of both insects, the female drops to the ground and finds a place to lay her thousands of eggs, thus starting a new generation.

---

10. Unfed nymph, 8 diameters.
11. Engorged females, natural size.
12. Unfed females, 8 diameters.
13. Unfed male, 8 diameters.
14. Engorged nymph, 8 diameters.
15. Engorged female, with eggs, natural size.

The life cycle of the tick is normally two years, but when food is extraordinarily scarce it may be extended to four years.

5.3 The Tick Control Program

During the 1909 season, Birdseye shot and trapped more than a thousand wild animals, from the smallest field mice to elk, bear, and mountain goats. King examined these animals for ticks, in order to determine the relative importance of each as a tick host. On the basis of their findings that season, King and Birdseye came to the conclusion that the tick family would soon die off or at least be greatly reduced, if grown ticks could be prevented from feeding and mating on cattle and horses, and if the immature forms were unable to find rodent hosts. They recommended dipping horses and cattle in oil to kill the adult ticks, and shooting and poisoning the ground squirrels to reduce the immature forms. This was the program that Ricketts had in mind before he died.

5.4 Geographic Range of *Dermacentor Andersoni*

Epidemiologic surveys conducted during the period 1909-1911 by the U.S. Bureau of Entomology revealed that the range of *Dermacentor andersoni* extends from the southern half of British Columbia and the western portions of Alberta to the northern edge of New Mexico.

5.5 U.S. Public Health Service Participation

In the spring of 1911, the U.S. Public Health Service sent Dr. Thomas B. McClintic to Montana to start a tick control program of dipping livestock and exterminating gophers (27). Because the Montana State Board of Health bypassed Dr. R. A. Cooley (28), the entomologist who had originally suggested the idea, considerable rivalry, animosity, and duplication of efforts resulted. As a direct consequence of this feud, a Montana State Board of Entomology was created in March, 1913. In 1912, Dr. McClintic contracted spotted fever in Montana and died on his way back to Washington. His death marked another tragedy of the spotted fever work.

5.6 Acceptance of the Control Program by Ranchers

Convincing the ranchers in the Bitter Root Valley of the efficacy of control measures was a difficult task requiring several years of patient diplomacy. By the end of the 1914 season the tick population of the Bitter Root had been enormously reduced, and there was an encouraging decrease in the number of cases of spotted fever. By the fall of 1915, even the most antagonistic residents were admitting that the control program was of benefit. Their animals were healthier and put on more weight when free of ticks.

5.7 The Sheep Lanolin Theory

Soon after Dr. McClintic's death in 1912, Dr. L. D. Fricks (29) arrived in Missoula to represent the U.S. Public Health Service. Although he participated in the dipping program he was looking for an easier and surer method of tick control. He believed that the lanolin in sheep's wool would kill ticks, and that the tick population could be decimated by turning sheep to graze on infected pastures. The first experiments conducted to test this hypothesis were inconclusive, but subsequent studies refuted the theory.

5.8 Participation of Ralph R. Parker

In 1916 Dr. Ralph R. Parker, another young entomologist, was employed by the Montana Board of
Entomology and began his studies on spotted fever—
studies which eventually led to the development of a
practical vaccine. While studying entomology at Massachusetts State College, Parker had spent several weeks at
Harvard University with Dr. S. Burt Wolbach, who was
then in the midst of studies on spotted fever. Parker
received his Ph.D. degree from Massachusetts State College in 1914. In 1916 he brought his bride from Smith
College to Powderville, Montana, where he spent his
honeymoon in a log cabin studying ticks (30). In May,
1917, Harold C. Urey (Nobel laureate in chemistry in
1934) arrived in Montana to assist Parker with his work.
The initial project was directed toward rodent control by
poisoning. By 1920 this program was so successful that
collecting ticks by dragging for four days on thirteen
ranches in the Stevensville area uncovered only eight
ticks. By this time stockmen had been convinced of the
efficacy of the control program and were completely
cooperative.

CHAPTER VI

Gross and Microscopic Pathologic Findings and Discovery Of the Etiologic Agent

6.1 Gross Pathologic Findings

By 1919 the literature contained reports of about fifteen autopsies performed on patients dying of spotted fever, all in the Bitter Root Valley (31). The early onset of intense rigor mortis was noted. The only constant distinctive findings on gross examination were the skin lesions and enlargement of the spleen, which weighed two to four times more than normal. The liver was usually large, pale, and injected, and often contained fat. The skin lesions found after death consisted of gangrene and hemorrhages into the subcutaneous tissues. The gross findings otherwise were essentially those of any infectious disease.

6.2 Microscopic Lesions

S. Burt Wolbach, M.D., professor of pathology at Harvard Medical School, was the first investigator to describe in detail the microscopic lesions of spotted fever (32). The characteristic findings he reported were focal lesions in the peripheral blood vessels and a general increase in large mononuclear phagocytes (endothelial

45

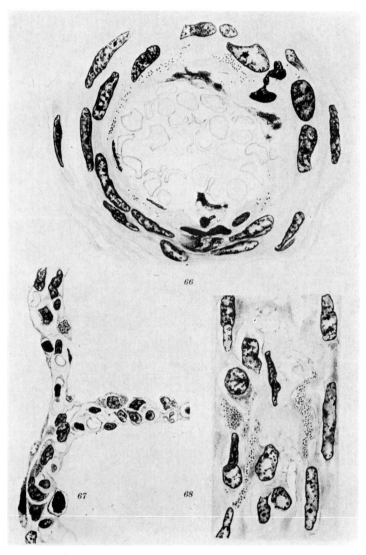

FIGURE 6. The pathologic anatomy of Rocky Mountain spotted fever.
66. Arteriole, skin of scrotum, human case. Giemsa's stain,

cells) in the capillaries of the various organs. These descriptions were based on five autopsies.

Both in man and in experimental animals the lesions of Rocky Mountain spotted fever are virtually restricted to the peripheral blood vessels, including those of the external genitalia. The vascular lesion is in the beginning a proliferative lesion of the endothelium. Since the reaction varies in intensity, polymorphonuclear leukocytes may or may not play a part in the lesions before thrombosis occurs; following thrombosis, polymorphonuclear cells are of necessity present. Evidence that the parasite directly injures cells is afforded by the degenerative changes found in the endothelium and in the smooth-muscle cells of the media, which are also invaded by the parasite. That the reaction to the disease is generalized is shown by the accumulations of endothelial cells in the lymph nodes and in the blood vessels of the lung, liver, and spleen.

One feature of Rocky Mountain spotted fever which cannot be too strongly emphasized is that the human disease can be exactly duplicated in experimental animals. In all mammals Rocky Mountain spotted fever is a disease of the peripheral blood vessels—an acute, specific infectious endangiitis.

6.3 Discovery of the Causative Agent of Rocky Mountain Spotted Fever

Although Wolbach (33) is generally credited with

---

showing distribution of the parasites and early reaction. 1,500 diameters.

67. Section through alveolar wall of lung to show the accumulation of endothelial cells. 750 diameters.

68. Parasites in smooth-muscle fibers in a tangentially-cut section of a testicular artery from a human case.

discovering the parasite of spotted fever in mammals, he himself believed that Ricketts most certainly had seen the organism in the blood of infected animals and man. He also believed that, in the tick, Ricketts had been misled by the presence of bacteria in the tissues.

Wolbach was convinced, from the pathologic nature of the lesion in the blood vessels, that the parasite must be present locally. He found the organism first with the eosin-methylene-blue stain in thin paraffin sections of zenkerized material. In these sections the parasite invariably had the form of a minute paired organism, often surrounded by a very narrow but definite clear zone, as if encapsulated. The length of the pair was approximately 1 micron, and the width 0.2 to 0.3 micron. This paired lanceolate form was found in the endothelial cells of the vascular lesions, being most abundant in smooth-muscle cells of the media. Individual smooth-muscle fibers were frequently found to be completely filled with the organisms. Smear preparations of mammalian tissues showed, in addition to the lanceolate organisms, slender rod-shaped forms, some of which had polar granules. The structural characteristics and the distribution of the parasite in the tissues were identical in all mammals studied: man, monkey, rabbit, and guinea pig.

Wolbach was convinced that the microorganism of Rocky Mountain spotted fever represented a new type of parasite. He proposed "the name *Dermacentroxenus rickettsi* for this organism in honor of Ricketts who first saw it in the blood" (33). Wolbach spent two years trying to cultivate the organism in vitro on every conceivable medium, including tissue culture, but was unsuccessful.

CHAPTER VII

The Vaccine

7.1 Status of the Spotted Fever Problem at the End of 1919

By the end of 1919, the causative agent of Rocky Mountain spotted fever had been identified but not yet cultured artificially. Small and large mammals had been identified as the natural reservoirs of infection. Much had been learned about the life cycle of *Dermacentor andersoni,* the only known vector of Rocky Mountain spotted fever, and the hereditary transmission of the organism in the tick was suspected. Man appeared to be an accidental host for the adult tick, and the peculiar occurrence of the disease in man had been explained on the basis of the habits of the tick in nature (34). The increase in the incidence of spotted fever in the Bitter Root Valley following its settlement by the white man was attributed to the introduction of large mammal hosts (cattle and horses) and the consequent increase in the population of infected ticks. Efforts to control the tick by eradicating small mammal hosts and by dipping cattle and horses had proved successful. Lacking still were a protective serum or vaccine and specific treatment for the disease.

7.2 Transmission by the Rabbit Tick

Ralph R. Parker, in 1921, showed that the rabbit tick,

49

Haemophysalis leporis palustris, not only can transmit the organism of spotted fever, but actually carries this organism in nature (35). After twenty-five years of study, it was finally learned that the wood tick is not the only vector.

7.3 Collaboration of R. R. Spencer and R. R. Parker

Federal participation in spotted fever research was increased in September, 1921, when Dr. R. R. Parker was employed by the U.S. Public Health Service to continue his studies on the disease. In the spring of 1922, Dr. R. R. Spencer, a staff member of the U.S. Public Health Service in Washington, was assigned to work with Dr. Parker in Montana. Popular demand for a vaccine to protect man from spotted fever was increasing.

7.4 Virulence Versus Immunity

At this time, the only way of determining whether a tick was infected was to allow it to feed on a guinea pig and await the development of typical clinical disease in the animal. Parker and Spencer conceived the idea of macerating pooled tick tissue and injecting it directly into guinea pigs. These experiments showed that ticks, when they first come out of hibernation, frequently contain the virus in a phase which produces only a low-grade infection. Such low-grade infections nevertheless immunized laboratory animals against spotted fever so that they were resistant to subsequent injections of infective material. This observation suggested that the ingestion of blood by overwintered adult ticks somehow changes the virus from a nonvirulent, immunity-producing phase to a virulent, fever-producing phase. Spencer now believed that a practical vaccine was possible (36).

7.5 The Spencer-Parker Vaccine

Spencer and Parker verified Ricketts' suggestion that infected female ticks can transmit the rickettsiae to the next generation through their eggs. They found that one such egg injected into a guinea pig is capable of producing spotted fever. Another finding was that ticks which become infected early in their life transmit a more highly fatal infection than ticks which become infected in adult life. Apparently the rickettsiae become more concentrated in ticks which carry them through several stages of growth.

In 1924, Parker found that a suspension of infected ticks which had been treated with phenol was protective for guinea pigs. The first human test with this material was performed by Spencer on himself. A sample of Spencer's blood before vaccination, mixed with virulent rickettsiae and injected into guinea pigs, did not protect them against spotted fever. His blood after vaccination, mixed with the same rickettsiae, protected guinea pigs from the disease.

The vaccine developed by Spencer and Parker was made from spotted fever rickettsiae obtained from infected ticks ("tick virus") rather than from the blood of infected animals. After its virulence was attenuated by chemical means, it was standardized for approximate potency by biologic (guinea pig) assay. Each dose (2 cc) was equivalent to 20,000 doses which would be minimally infectious for a guinea pig. Two such doses at five-day intervals constituted the standard course, which had to be repeated annually. Equally good protection was afforded by subcutaneous, intravenous, intramuscular, and intraperitoneal routes (the last usually being employed only in guinea pigs). Ordinarily, the material was administered subcutaneously.

7.6 Manufacture of the Vaccine

The original vaccine was quite expensive, costing $20 per injection. Efforts were next devoted to producing this material in large quantities. Wild adult ticks, collected in the field, were allowed to feed on infected guinea pigs after the onset of the fever. After two days of feeding, the ticks were removed and stored for several months. Before being used for making vaccine, these ticks were again fed, this time on normal animals for five or six days. After this second feeding, which produced a marked increase in the concentration of the virus, the partly engorged ticks were ground with a mortar and pestle, and a preservative of 1.6 per cent phenol and 0.4 per cent formalin was added. The vaccine was made from the supernate of the suspension. Vaccine production was obviously a tedious, expensive, and dangerous work. In the spring of 1925 the supply was adequate only to vaccinate thirty-four persons in the Bitter Root Valley (37).

7.7 The First Vaccination Program

In 1926 a vaccination program was carried out in the Bitter Root Valley and in Idaho. In the Bitter Root, vaccination greatly diminished the mortality of the virulent type of spotted fever and also shortened the period of illness (38). In Idaho one case of spotted fever developed in the vaccinated group, while twenty-two cases occurred in an equal number of unvaccinated volunteers. The vaccine's value was evident. It prevented the occurrence of the mild type of spotted fever and reduced the mortality in the highly fatal type of the disease from about 85 per cent to about 10 per cent.

Partly as a result of these successes, the state legislature of Montana, in 1927, was requested to finance a new building for the State Board of Entomology. Hamilton was chosen as the site, and the Montana Research Laboratory came into existence in 1928.

7.8 Establishment of the Rocky Mountain Research Laboratory

The demand for the spotted fever vaccine increased so rapidly that it was no longer feasible to make it from wild ticks. In the Montana Research Laboratory the cultivation of ticks on a large scale was initiated. At peak production more than a million infected ticks a year were cultivated for the vaccine—an enterprise requiring 15,000 to 20,000 guinea pigs and 6,000 rabbits.

Even as the supply of vaccine increased, Rocky Mountain spotted fever spread and became a major problem in several other western states besides Montana and Idaho. By 1930, the demand for the vaccine exceeded the production capacity of the Montana Research Laboratory, and it appeared reasonable that other states should share in financing the activities of this laboratory. The logical solution was for the federal government to buy the laboratory from the state. In February, 1932, the Montana Research Laboratory at Hamilton was sold by the state to the federal government and became the Rocky Mountain Research Laboratory of Hamilton, Montana, a part of the U. S. Public Health Service. Production of vaccine continued there and, in 1948, enough vaccine for 140,000 persons was produced at a cost of $1.00 per injection.

7.9 Results of Long-term Studies with the Vaccine

Less than 5 per cent of 4,000 persons vaccinated complained of constitutional symptoms (39). These included malaise, slight fever, nausea, and aching joints or muscles. Serum sickness, with urticaria and edema, occurred in 1 per cent of the recipients. Local reactions were mostly inconsequential, being limited usually to local redness, swelling, and itching about the site of injection.

Data from the Bitter Root Valley tests showed that protection usually does not extend beyond one tick season. Hence, annual vaccination was recommended (40).

Three lots of the Spencer-Parker vaccine manufactured in 1928 and 1929 were stored at a temperature of 34° to 40° F. and retested for potency in March, 1942. Their protective values appeared to be undiminished. This test indicated that the vaccine is good for at least twelve to fourteen years (41).

7.10 The Noguchi Serovaccine

An interesting sidelight is that Dr. Hideo Noguchi, of the Rockefeller Institute in New York, early in 1923 announced the development of a serovaccine, containing immune serum and the organism (42). Noguchi had received from Parker several strains of the spotted fever organism and had used them in a systematic study on the phenomenon of immunity in spotted fever. He had found his serovaccine to be effective in protecting guinea pigs against spotted fever, but had not yet tried it on human beings.

Noguchi was invited to appear at a conference held in Missoula on April 5 and 6, 1923. Here he presented a paper entitled "Prophylactic Inoculation against Rocky

Mountain Spotted Fever" (43), and asked for volunteers to take his serum, which he himself refused to take. Since he was a Japanese, the management of the Northern Pacific Railroad brought nine of their Japanese workers to meet him, and Noguchi persuaded them to be inoculated. The railroad offered its hospital facilities for any who experienced severe reactions. The serum was given in two doses a week apart, and severe serum sickness did indeed develop in several of the recipients. In deference to the fame of Noguchi, Spencer and Parker remained quiet and continued with their own efforts to develop a safe and effective vaccine.

7.11 The Honor Role

By 1928, the honor role of martyrs in the fight against spotted fever read as follows:

Dr. Howard T. Ricketts, 1910
Dr. Thomas B. McClintic, U.S.P.H.S., 1912
William E. Gittinger, U.S.P.H.S., 1922
George H. Cowan, field worker with the
Montana State Board of Entomology, 1922
Arthur LeRoy Kerlee, U.S.P.H.S., 1928

CHAPTER VIII

The Recognition of Spotted Fever in the East

8.1 Spotted Fever in the Western and Mountain States

By the early 1930s, as the curse of spotted fever on the Bitter Root Valley was being lifted by the success of the tick-control and vaccination programs, the disease had spread or was being recognized elsewhere. During the nineteen-twenties, it became a custom with stockmen in Wyoming and Montana to fatten their cattle in feed lots. Two cases of spotted fever occurred in Chadron, Nebraska, in 1930 and were reported almost apologetically by Pierce and Vanderkamp (44). Both patients recovered. By 1931, spotted fever had been officially reported from the states of California, Colorado, North and South Dakota, Nebraska, Nevada, Oregon, Utah, Washington, and Wyoming. The outbreaks in these infected states were rather sharply localized in certain small areas.

8.2 Transmission by the Wood, Rabbit, and Dog Ticks

At this time it was still generally believed that Rocky Mountain spotted fever was transmitted to human beings solely by the bite of an infected adult wood tick, *Dermacentor andersoni*. It will be recalled, however, that Parker in 1923 had reported the transmission of rickettsiae in the life cycle of the rabbit tick, *Haemaphysalis leporis*

palustris (35). As early as 1911, Maver (45), a col-
laborator of Ricketts, had reported the transmission of
spotted fever by the American dog tick, *Dermacentor
variabilis*. In July, 1909, Dr. Ricketts himself had collected specimens of this tick in the vicinity of Woods
Hole, Massachusetts. Maver had also shown that *Dermacentor marginatus* and *Amblyoma americanum*, the "Lone
Star tick," could be infected and later transmit the
infection. It was logical to anticipate that spotted fever
could occur wherever these ticks resided.

8.3 Endemic Typhus Fever or Spotted Fever?

In the early nineteen-thirties there began to appear in
the states of the Eastern Seaboard an endemic disease
which resembled the typhus fever of Europe. The fatality
rate in 1930 was about 23 per cent. The U.S. Public
Health Service was extremely interested in this problem.
Dyer, Rumreich, and Badger (46) noted that many of
the cases observed in the spring and summer of 1930
closely resembled Rocky Mountain spotted fever.

Unlike true endemic typhus, which is predominantly of
urban origin, these exanthems occurred in persons living
in rural sections or having rural contacts. In a high
percentage of cases the illness was preceded by a tick
bite; in occasional cases where there was no history of
tick bite, the patients had crushed engorged ticks removed
from domestic animals. The clinical symptoms and signs
were typical of mild to moderately severe Rocky Mountain spotted fever.

Blood drawn from these patients and injected into
laboratory animals produced a disease which Badger
found to be identical with spotted fever in all particulars,
except that it was less severe and lacked the scrotal

inflammation which characterized the virulent Montana strain. Complete cross-immunity between the Eastern and Western strains was demonstrated.

Highly virulent strains of rickettsiae were subsequently isolated from *D. variabilis* in many Eastern and Southern states (47, 48); when these organisms were injected into guinea pigs, the scrotal lesions and other signs commonly associated with the Bitter Root (Western) strain of spotted fever appeared after the usual short incubation period.

8.4 Pathologic Findings in the Eastern Type

Lillie (49) found that bronchopneumonia, which is relatively infrequent in the Western form of spotted fever, was present in most of the patients who succumbed to the Eastern type. Other distinctive pathologic features of the latter variety are less marked splenomegaly, the absence of scrotal gangrene and of ecchymoses in the serous membranes, and the presence of focal degenerative and proliferative vascular lesions, as well as focal gliosis, in the brain. Arteriolar "thrombonecroses" with surrounding infarctions were found in the heart, gastrointestinal tract, skin and loose connective tissues, pancreas, kidneys, urinary bladder, spinal cord, and to some extent in the lungs, as well as in the brain. The reticuloendothelial system was hyperplastic (50).

8.5 Transmission of Rickettsiae by the Dog Tick

The disease first reported as endemic typhus was finally identified as an Eastern type of Rocky Mountain spotted fever, transmitted by the common dog tick, *D. variabilis*. These ticks were experimentally infected in the laboratory by allowing them to feed, as larvae, on infected guinea pigs. After these larvae had molted, the organisms were recovered from the nymphs (51). Rickettsiae were also demonstrated in dog ticks obtained from a farm in Virginia on which a human case of spotted fever had occurred (52). It was then learned that dogs themselves are susceptible to spotted fever. Fever and respiratory symptoms developed in dogs inoculated with the spotted fever organism, and rickettsiae were recovered from their blood (53).

8.6 Range and Danger of the Dog Tick

As early as 1912, it was known that the dog tick occurs east and south of a line starting just west of the southern-most tip of Texas and extending northward and eastward across the states of Oklahoma, Kansas, Missouri, Illinois, and Indiana into southern Michigan, and thence almost due east across northern New York and the southern portions of Vermont, New Hampshire, and Maine.

In some respects the dog tick is a more dangerous vector of spotted fever than the wood tick. It is active from spring until fall, and the larvae and nymphs which bite man so freely are abundant in the late summer and early fall, when the adult wood ticks are decreasing in number. Since the hosts of *D. variabilis* are mainly domesticated animals such as the dog, horse, and cow, tick infestation may be greater about the areas of habitation. Because dogs are so often household pets, a high percentage of infections in the East occur among children.

8.7 The Disease in Other States and Countries

In 1933, Parker, Philip, and Jellison of the Rocky Mountain Laboratory (54) reported the occurrence of a possible case of spotted fever in Maryland in 1926, a definite case in Missouri in 1931, and four cases in Louisiana in 1931. All the evidence suggested that the dog tick was the vector of the disease in each of these cases. Cumming (55) estimated that in 1933 not less than 500 cases had occurred in the Western states and at least 200 had been reported in the rest of the country.

No further evidence definitely incriminating the dog tick appeared until late in August, 1941, when spotted fever broke out in Oklahoma and Texas. In Oklahoma, six members of a single family were stricken within a month; all had been bitten by dog ticks on their own premises. Moreover, the attending physician, who spent a night with the family, also contracted spotted fever. Nymphs of *D. variabilis* and pocket gophers trapped on the premises contained strains of spotted fever rickettsiae, which were later isolated in guinea pigs (56).

During the next few years, spotted fever was reported from New York, Pennsylvania, Maryland, Virginia, Delaware, New Jersey, North Carolina, South Carolina, Georgia, Tennessee, Texas, Louisiana, Oklahoma, and the District of Columbia. By 1948 the only states in the union in which spotted fever had not been reported were Maine, Vermont, Rhode Island, Connecticut, Michigan, and Kansas.

Rocky Mountain spotted fever was first recognized in Brazil by Piza in 1931 (57), in Colombia by Patino in 1937 (58), in Canada by Hearle in 1938 (59), in Mexico by Bustamente and Varela in 1943 (60), and in Panama by De Rodaniche and Rodaniche in 1950 (61).

CHAPTER IX

Artificial Cultivation of the Rickettsia of Spotted Fever

9.1 Histologic Evidences for a Specific Microorganism

Ricketts was probably the first investigator to see the organism of spotted fever (19), and Wolbach was the first to describe it in detail (32). It was Wolbach who gave it the name *Dermacentroxenus rickettsi*. By 1919 the following histologic evidences left no doubt that this was the causative agent of Rocky Mountain spotted fever: (1) The constant occurrence of a microorganism of distinctive size and structure in the lesions which characterized the disease in man, monkey, rabbit, and guinea pig; (2) the constant presence in infective ticks of an identical organism showing undoubted evidences of developmental phases, and the absence of this organism in noninfective ticks; (3) the recognition of this specific organism in the tissues and eggs of infected ticks.

9.2 Tissue Culture

The organism identified histologically as the causative agent of spotted fever proved impossible to cultivate on artificial or cell-free media. After numerous failures, Wolbach and his coworkers finally succeeded in growing the microorganism in cultures of tissue and plasma (62, 63). The successful propagation of *D. rickettsi* in tissue

61

culture proved beyond a doubt that the etiologic agent
of Rocky Mountain spotted fever is a living microorganism.

That the parasites go through a developmental cycle
in ticks was recognized by Wolbach, who described three
morphologic types observed in tissue cultures: (1) a
relatively large extranuclear bacillus-like form, without
chromatoid granules, and present in ticks only during the
initial multiplication of the parasites; (2) a relatively
small rod-shaped form with chromatoid granules, which
is probably the same form seen within nuclei in sections
of ticks, and rarely in smooth-muscle cells in the blood
vessels of mammals, and (3) a relatively large, lanceolate,
paired form, present in ticks and in blood and lesions
from infected mammals.

9.3 Cultivation in the Developing Chick Embryo

Further success in the artificial cultivation of rickettsiae
was a direct result of efforts to produce more efficiently
a spotted fever vaccine in larger volume, and with less
risk to personnel. By 1935, there was no evidence that
the agent of spotted fever could be propagated in media
which did not contain living elements. Only two choices
of methods were available: tissue culture and cultivation
in the developing chick embryo. The method of tissue
culture employed at that time, however, presented so
many technical difficulties that it could not be utilized
for vaccine production.

The first investigators to appreciate the value of the
developing chick embryo for the experimental study of
a viral agent were Rous and Murphy (64), who used
this medium prior to 1911 to grow the virus of chicken
sarcoma No. 1 (Rous sarcoma). Major credit today,

however, is given to Goodpasture and his associates (65) for first emphasizing (in 1931) the tremendous possibilities in the use of developing chick embryos for "research work and in practical applications to prevention and treatment."

In 1935 Bengtson and Dyer (66) used the techniques of Goodpasture to cultivate the rickettsiae of spotted fever on the chorioallantoic membrane of chick embryos ten to twelve days old. The original inoculum, consisting of a saline suspension of emulsified spleen from an infected guinea pig, was dropped on the surface of the chorioallantoic membrane and the eggs were incubated at 33° C. Death of the embryo occurred regularly on the fifth or sixth day, and a characteristic lesion—a small, discrete, cloudy area—was found at the site of inoculation. Histologic examination of these lesions revealed focal perivascular or interstitial infiltration by lymphocytes in the fetal membranes, skin, skeletal muscle, meso- and meta-nephroi, heart muscle, liver, meninges, and other organs. Confined to the fetal membranes were foci of vascular endothelial swelling, eccentric adventitial fibroblastic proliferation, and occasional vascular thrombonecrosis (67).

In the chorioallantoic membrane, the rickettsiae were demonstrated characteristically in the cytoplasm of the epithelial cells, frequently in a peripheral position; no rickettsiae were observed within nuclei. This membrane, when inoculated into guinea pigs, almost invariably produced symptoms of Rocky Mountain spotted fever. The infective dose for guinea pigs was about 1 cc of the 1:10,000 dilution of an entire infected membrane. The organism was present also in the brain and liver of the embryo but at a lower concentration.

9.4 The Yolk-Sac Method

In 1936 Dr. Herald R. Cox was added to the staff of the Rocky Mountain Laboratory at Hamilton, Montana, for the express purpose of finding a simple method of producing spotted fever vaccine. After about two years of unsuccessful efforts, he tried embryonated chick eggs. Growth of rickettsiae occurred most luxuriantly in the yolk-sac membrane (68) of eggs incubated at 35° C; the rickettsiae continued to grow if the eggs were kept at room temperature (20 to 22° C) for two or three days after the death of the embryo (69). The yolk sac was found to be more infectious than any other tissue. The yolk-sac suspension was 100 to 1,000 times more infectious than any other material then available, and was so virulent that dilutions of 1:1,000,000 produced clinical disease in guinea pigs.

9.5 Routine Method for Production of Vaccine

The yolk-sac method for the production of spotted fever vaccine was as follows: The yolk sacs of fertile chick eggs were inoculated with the rickettsiae, and the eggs were incubated for a few days at 32° C. The yolk sacs were then removed, pooled, and ground. After the rickettsiae were killed chemically and the fat was extracted, the resultant material was the vaccine.

The features which made this technique particularly valuable were its extreme simplicity and the ease with which the cultures could be maintained with a minimal risk of contamination. During one year, Cox used thirty dozen eggs daily and found contaminants in less than one egg per 2,500.

A bacteriologist and two assistants could now prepare forty to fifty liters of vaccine weekly. The material from twenty eggs was sufficient for approximately one liter of vaccine. It became feasible at Hamilton to prepare the vaccine in lots of twenty-five to thirty-five liters each. The same general technique was applicable to the production of vaccine for European and endemic typhus and for "Q" fever. The problem of vaccine production had been solved.

9.6 Antigenicity of Chick Vaccine

None of the individuals vaccinated with this new type of vaccine reported any reaction other than slight local tenderness at the site of inoculation; this always disappeared within a day or so. The evidence suggested that the chick vaccine was more easily tolerated than the tick type. No untoward reactions were observed in a number of persons known to be allergic to egg protein.

9.7 Purification of Rickettsiae

The abundant growth of the rickettsiae in the yolk sac made it possible to prepare, by fractional centrifugation methods, practically pure suspensions of rickettsiae suitable for agglutination tests. The possibility of using such pure material for diagnostic skin tests was entertained.

9.8 Establishment of an Avirulent Strain

The yolk-sac technique was also employed in the establishment of an avirulent strain of *D. rickettsi* which produced, in guinea pigs, solid immunity to massive doses of highly virulent strains. The relative merits of this vaccine as opposed to the vaccine made from killed organisms remain to be ascertained.

9.9 Factors Influencing Growth of Rickettsiae

Greiff, Pinkerton, and Moragues (70) have reported that sodium fluoride seems to accelerate the growth of rickettsiae in the yolk sac, and have suggested that this agent may render the entodermal cells of the yolk sac more susceptible to infection by certain disease-producing agents.

Cox (71) found in 1942 that a technique using both living and dead embryos can be used to increase the yield of tissue infected with spotted fever. When seven-day embryos were inoculated in the yolk sac and then incubated at 32 to 36° C, they died within three or four days. At this time the concentration of rickettsiae in the yolk sac yielded approximately a million infecting doses per gram of tissue, whereas the chorioallantoic membrane contained relatively few rickettsiae. If eggs were kept at room temperature for two to four days after death of the embryos, however, the rickettsiae continued to grow, particularly in the chorioallantoic membrane, until this tissue showed a concentration approximately equivalent to that found in the yolk sac. There is need for further study on the relationship between the growth of rickettsiae and the metabolism and viability of cells.

Of interest in this regard is Pinkerton's (72) observation that a temperature of 32° C is optimal for the extracellular growth of both typhus and spotted fever rickettsiae. At this temperature, he was able to establish and maintain for an indefinite period cultures in which practically every cell was packed with microorganisms by about the fourteenth day of incubation. During mitosis the rickettsiae diminished in number; those that remained assumed a globular form and were found in the periphery of cells—away from the region of the dividing chromosomes. This finding suggests that the process of mitosis is temporarily unfavorable to the organism. Pinkerton suggested that the rate of cellular metabolism may be an important factor in rickettsial infections, a high rate enabling the cell to free itself from the intracellular parasites.

In cultures of guinea-pig tissue incubated at 32° C, the rickettsiae were confined to the interior of cells and were never seen in the plasma clot (72). The outstanding feature of these cultures was the predilection of spotted fever rickettsiae for the nuclei of cells, although infection of the cytoplasm without nuclear involvement was also seen in many cases. Although Wolbach (32) had described intranuclear rickettsiae in tick tissue, Pinkerton and Hass (73) were the first to describe the intranuclear location of spotted fever rickettsiae (or, for that matter, of any microorganism) in mammalian tissues. No good explanation has been offered for the clustering of rickettsiae within nuclei, in contrast to their apparently diffuse distribution in the cytoplasm of cells.

9.10 Morphologic Characteristics of Rickettsiae

The rickettsiae as a group may be characterized as follows: small, often pleomorphic, bacterium-like microorganisms, living and multiplying in arthropod tissues, not cultivable in any known cell-free medium, usually behaving as obligate intracellular parasites, and staining lightly with aniline dyes. Rickettsiae vary considerably in their structure, ranging from minute coccoid bodies about 0.2 micron in greatest dimension to long threads (mostly chains of bacilli) up to 0.8 micron in diameter and 15 microns in length. The thread forms are much more frequent in the cytoplasm, and smaller bacillary and coccoid forms appear in the nucleus (73).

CHAPTER X

Diagnostic and Immunologic Studies on Spotted Fever

10.1 Clinical Diagnosis

Although classic Rocky Mountain spotted fever presents an easily recognizable clinical picture, the very mild infections and the rapidly fulminating cases may be quite difficult to diagnose. This disease should be suspected whenever a febrile illness occurs during the tick season in a person exposed to ticks. Careful examination may reveal a tick still attached, or an indurated area suggesting the site of a tick bite. In the Eastern states, careful inspection of the scalp is important, especially in young girls with long hair.

The differential diagnosis may be difficult, particularly in areas where spotted fever and endemic typhus are both prevalent. The symptoms at onset may resemble those of a severe cold or influenza. After the rash appears, other exanthems such as measles and endemic typhus must be considered. Less frequently, spotted fever may be confused with meningococcal meningitis, typhoid fever and allied conditions, smallpox, purpura, erythema nodosum, Colorado tick fever, brucellosis, encephalitis, and streptococcal septicemia. When confusion does exist, the correct diagnosis usually becomes apparent clinically as the disease progresses. If not, the diagnosis can be established in the laboratory unless the disease is rapidly fatal. The laboratory procedures ordinarily used for diagnosis are the infection test, the Weil-Felix reaction, the protection or virus neutralization test, and the complement-fixation test.

It should be emphasized that no laboratory procedure is consistently reliable in making the diagnosis of Rocky Mountain spotted fever during the first week or ten days of the illness. During this phase, a high index of suspicion on the part of the physician, a history of recent exposure to ticks, and an accurate evaluation of the clinical manifestations, especially the rash, are of paramount importance in making a diagnosis.

10.2 The Infection Test

The infection test is the original method used by Ricketts (11) in 1906 to transfer the infection from man to guinea pig. Male guinea pigs are inoculated intraperitoneally with blood from a suspected case. Clotted blood, plasma, or serum may be used, but citrated whole blood is preferable. If the test is positive, the animals begin to have fever and swelling of the testicles and scrotum within a few days; hemorrhages into the skin of the scrotum soon follow.

Once the disease is established, it can be maintained by the intraperitoneal inoculation of normal male guinea pigs with blood, splenic tissue, or testicular washings taken from an infected guinea pig on the second or third day of fever. Maintaining the infection in guinea pigs makes it possible to apply cross-immunity tests with known strains of spotted fever rickettsiae and other infectious agents.

disease, the Weil-Felix test cannot be used for epidemiologic studies of past infections in a given area.

When the Weil-Felix test is used, it is desirable to
obtain at least two blood samples: one as soon as spotted
fever is suspected, the other approximately two weeks
after the onset. The first blood sample is seldom diagnostic and is valuable chiefly as a reference point for
ascertaining whether the second specimen shows a rise
in titer. A titer of at least 1:320 must be attained for
the test to be definitely diagnostic.

10.4 The Protection or Virus-neutralization Test

According to Parker (85), the protection or virus-
neutralization test is nearly always of diagnostic value.
To three samples of the patient's serum (0.5 cc each)
are added 0.1, 0.25, and 0.5 cc of blood from guinea pigs
infected with spotted fever. After being held at room
temperature for thirty minutes, the mixtures are injected
intraperitoneally into guinea pigs. Control animals receive
the same amount of infectious guinea pig serum mixed
with normal serum. Animals injected with serum from
patients who have antibodies to spotted fever do not
develop the disease; control animals develop the typical
signs. This neutralization test is claimed to be of greater
value than the infection test.

10.5 The Preparation of a Pure, Specific Antigen

Numerous investigators, aware of the many limitations
of the Weil-Felix reaction, attempted to develop specific
rickettsial antigens for use in immunologic tests. The
chief obstacle was overcome when Cox (68) introduced
the yolk-sac culture method, by which pure suspensions
of rickettsiae could be prepared in amounts sufficient to
be of general use. Bengtson (86) used this method to

established in the laboratory unless the disease is rapidly fatal. The laboratory procedures ordinarily used for diagnosis are the infection test, the Weil-Felix reaction, the protection or virus neutralization test, and the complement-fixation test.

It should be emphasized that no laboratory procedure is consistently reliable in making the diagnosis of Rocky Mountain spotted fever during the first week or ten days of the illness. During this phase, a high index of suspicion on the part of the physician, a history of recent exposure to ticks, and an accurate evaluation of the clinical manifestations, especially the rash, are of paramount importance in making a diagnosis.

10.2 The Infection Test

The infection test is the original method used by Ricketts (11) in 1906 to transfer the infection from man to guinea pig. Male guinea pigs are inoculated intraperitoneally with blood from a suspected case. Clotted blood, plasma, or serum may be used, but citrated whole blood is preferable. If the test is positive, the animals begin to have fever and swelling of the testicles and scrotum within a few days; hemorrhages into the skin of the scrotum soon follow.

Once the disease is established, it can be maintained by the intraperitoneal inoculation of normal male guinea pigs with blood, splenic tissue, or testicular washings taken from an infected guinea pig on the second or third day of fever. Maintaining the infection in guinea pigs makes it possible to apply cross-immunity tests with known strains of spotted fever rickettsiae and other infectious agents.

10.3 The Weil-Felix Reaction

When the clinical manifestations of Rocky Mountain spotted fever are not diagnostic and laboratory facilities and experimental animals are not available, serologic tests may be of great diagnostic aid.

For many years the only serologic test available for the detection of rickettsial infection was the Weil-Felix agglutination reaction, which tests the ability of the patient's serum to agglutinate *Proteus* organisms (76).

In 1916, Felix (77) isolated a strain of *Proteus vulgaris* from the urine of a patient with epidemic typhus fever. In studying the forms of dissociation, he recognized two types: a motile, flagellated type (H), and a nonmotile, unflagellated type (O). In animals inoculated with these two forms of the organisms, two type of agglutinins, differing in their antigenic structure, were produced. The *flagellar* (H) agglutinins were often found in the sera of patients with nonrickettsial diseases (particularly those due to *P. vulgaris*), or with a history of rickettsial diseases. The *somatic* (O) agglutinins, on the other hand, were found only in the blood of patients with typhus fever.

The O strains of *P. vulgaris*, therefore, are used in the diagnosis of the rickettsial group of diseases. Certain strains of *P. vulgaris*, especially those designated as OX-19, OX-2, and OX-K, have been found to be most useful in the diagnosis of rickettsial diseases.

After Felix (77) demonstrated the significance of the *Proteus* agglutination test in epidemic typhus, sera of patients with Rocky Mountain spotted fever were tested against the *Proteus OX-19* strain by Kelly (78) and by Kerlee and Spencer (79). Kelly obtained negative results, but Kerlee and Spencer found agglutinins and, in one case, a rise in antibody titer. Munter (80) found that the injection of spotted fever rickettsiae into rabbits produced agglutinins for *Proteus OX-19*. In subsequent studies (81-84), agglutinins for the *Proteus OX-2* strain were also demonstrated in the sera of human cases of spotted fever.

The usual Weil-Felix reaction in spotted fever (found by Plotz (84) in 70 per cent of the cases) is a high titer for *Proteus OX-19*, a lower titer or negative agglutination test with the *OX-2* strain, and a negative reaction with *OX-K*. In these cases the *OX-19* titer may reach levels equal to those found in either epidemic or murine typhus fever. The second most frequent combination, seen in 21 per cent of the cases reported by Plotz (84), is a high *Proteus OX-2* titer and a lower titer or negative reaction with *OX-19* and *OX-K*.

The Weil-Felix reaction is nonspecific and depends upon the presence of an antigenic fraction which is common to the Proteus organism and the rickettsiae. Hence it is impossible to differentiate epidemic typhus, murine typhus, and Rocky Mountain spotted fever by the Weil-Felix technique, since high titers for *Proteus OX-19* agglutinins appear in all three diseases. Positive reactions have been obtained in patients with nonrickettsial diseases.

Although the *Proteus* agglutinins usually appear toward the end of the second week of Rocky Mountain spotted fever, they are sometimes not present until early convalescence; some patients, in fact, never produce *Proteus* agglutinins. The Weil-Felix reaction usually becomes positive a few days before the appearance of complement-fixing antibodies. Since the *Proteus* agglutinins disappear in the late convalescence of patients with rickettsial

disease, the Weil-Felix test cannot be used for epidemiologic studies of past infections in a given area.

When the Weil-Felix test is used, it is desirable to
obtain at least two blood samples: one as soon as spotted
fever is suspected, the other approximately two weeks
after the onset. The first blood sample is seldom diagnostic and is valuable chiefly as a reference point for
ascertaining whether the second specimen shows a rise
in titer. A titer of at least 1:320 must be attained for
the test to be definitely diagnostic.

10.4 The Protection or Virus-neutralization Test

According to Parker (85), the protection or virus-
neutralization test is nearly always of diagnostic value.
To three samples of the patient's serum (0.5 cc each)
are added 0.1, 0.25, and 0.5 cc of blood from guinea pigs
infected with spotted fever. After being held at room
temperature for thirty minutes, the mixtures are injected
intraperitoneally into guinea pigs. Control animals receive
the same amount of infectious guinea pig serum mixed
with normal serum. Animals injected with serum from
patients who have antibodies to spotted fever do not
develop the disease; control animals develop the typical
signs. This neutralization test is claimed to be of greater
value than the infection test.

10.5 The Preparation of a Pure, Specific Antigen

Numerous investigators, aware of the many limitations
of the Weil-Felix reaction, attempted to develop specific
rickettsial antigens for use in immunologic tests. The
chief obstacle was overcome when Cox (68) introduced
the yolk-sac culture method, by which pure suspensions
of rickettsiae could be prepared in amounts sufficient to
be of general use. Bengtson (86) used this method to

prepare antigens with which she successfully performed complement-fixation tests upon sera from cases of murine typhus. Craigie (87) then succeeded in separating rickettsiae from yolk-sac suspensions by ether extraction, thereby eliminating most of the embryonic egg materials and making available essentially pure suspensions of rickettsiae for use as antigens in vaccines and serologic tests.

10.6 The Complement-fixation (C-F) Test

The chief advantage of the complement-fixation (C-F) test, as compared to the Weil-Felix reaction, is its specificity. The antigen first used for this test (prepared from the serum or macerated organs of infected guinea pigs and from infected tick eggs) gave unsatisfactory results, probably because it contained such small numbers of rickettsiae (88, 89). Antigen was next prepared from tissue cultures grown on semisolid agar (90); complement-fixing antibody was demonstrated in one serum specimen obtained from a patient with spotted fever on the twelfth day of illness, and it was also present in another specimen obtained four and a half years after the illness. Complement-fixing antigen is now usually prepared from yolk-sac material.

Complement-fixing antibodies may appear within eleven days after the onset of the clinical illness (91). The titer begins to fall after about six months, but the antibody may be detectable for six to eight years.

The C-F test, using purified rickettsial suspensions as antibodies, was recommended as a routine test for differentiating rickettsial infections (murine and epidemic typhus and Rocky Mountain spotted fever) in guinea pigs (92). Clinically, the C-F test appears to be a little more

specific for Rocky Mountain spotted fever than for
endemic typhus (93).

10.7 The Agglutination Reaction and Protection Test

Although Ricketts obtained specific agglutination reactions with suspensions of rickettsial organisms in 1909,
extensive work on this method was delayed by the lack
of pure antigenic material. In 1941, Fitzpatrick and
Hampil introduced the agglutination test as a diagnostic
method for the detection of antibodies (94). A culture
grown in chick embryos was used as antigen. The test
was performed by adding antigen to the serum dilutions
in hanging-drop slides, and incubating the slides for four
hours at 40° C.

The results were compared to those obtained with a
protection test in which 1 ml of guinea-pig blood containing virulent rickettsiae was mixed with varying
amounts of rabbit serum being tested for the presence
of the protective material. After being stored in an ice
box for several weeks, the mixtures were injected intraperitoneally into guinea pigs.

In rabbits experimentally infected with Rocky Mountain spotted fever, the sequence of appearance of
antibodies was as follows: the rickettsial agglutinins
appeared between the fifth and the eighth day after the
first injection of rickettsiae; the *proteus* agglutinins
between the seventh and the fourteenth day. The protective antibodies appeared last, at a time when the
rabbit blood was no longer infectious for guinea pigs.
In some of the rabbits a Weil-Felix reaction did not
develop, but this absence of Proteus agglutinins did not
affect the development of rickettsial agglutinins and
protective antibodies. Even in animals which continued

to receive injections of rickettsiae, the Weil-Felix reaction dropped to zero within one to five weeks. The rickettsial agglutinins and protective antibodies, on the other hand, persisted for as long as seven months.

10.8 The Soluble Antigen

In 1943 Castaneda (95) found that the agglutination of *Proteus* organisms by convalescent typhus serum could be explained on the basis of an antigen common to the rickettsiae and the *Proteus* bacillus. He reported that this material was a specific, soluble substance, probably a polysaccharide. Cohen and Chargaff (96), in 1944, found it to be a protein-carbohydrate conjugate of high molecular weight which possesses a distinctive chemical constitution. They postulated that it might be a product of rickettsial degradation, created either by proteolytic action or by the treatment employed during the purification of rickettsiae.

A year later Topping and Shear (97), in the process of preparing spotted fever antigen from infected yolk-sac material, found a soluble antigen in the supernatant fluid obtained after ether extraction and centrifugation. Complement was fixed to a higher degree by this fluid than by the rickettsial sediment. The antigen remained in the supernatant fluid after centrifugation at 15,000 rpm for fifteen minutes, and was not completely removed by filtration through a Berkefeld N filter. It was relatively stable to heat. When injected into rabbits, it induced a Weil-Felix reaction comparable to that produced by an alcoholic extract of the *Proteus* organism (presumably a carbohydrate fraction). Complement-fixing antibodies developed in guinea pigs inoculated with the soluble antigen, and these animals were immune on challenge with virulent rickettsiae; whether injection of the alcoholic extract of the *Proteus* organism can confer immunity against spotted fever is not known. In complement-fixation and precipitins test the soluble antigen, unlike washed rickettsiae, reacts with *Proteus OX-19* antisera.

Upon standing at 40° C, rickettsial suspensions devoid of free soluble antigen slowly become nonspecific immunologically; at the same time soluble antigen can be demonstrated in the supernatant fluid. This antigen can again be rendered specific by washing (98).

The serum of rabbits hyperimmunized with soluble antigen gives a positive Weil-Felix reaction, and contains complement-fixing antibodies and precipitins to the soluble antigen. The serum of rabbits inoculated with washed rickettsiae, on the other hand, contains rickettsial agglutinins and complement-fixing antibodies to washed rickettsiae, but does not give a Weil-Felix reaction.

Conclusive proof of the origin of this soluble antigen had to await the development of the electron microscope (99). Under this microscope, untreated rickettsiae show definite capsules, which are broken into shreds and droplets by the addition of ether. Although these droplets contain no rickettsial organisms, the addition of antiserum causes them to agglutinate. Thus it has been shown that the soluble antigen which has an antigenic structure common to the *Proteus* organism is the capsular material of the rickettsiae.

10.9 The Toxin

In 1953 Bell and Pickens (100) found, in yolk sacs infected with many strains of the spotted fever group of rickettsiae, specific toxic substances which were lethal to mice. This toxin was neutralized in relatively high titer by sera from human beings and guinea pigs convalescent from spotted fever, but was not neutralized by serum from normal human beings or guinea pigs, or by serum from guinea pigs previously infected with epidemic typhus, murine typhus, or Q fever. This toxin was also neutralized by sera obtained from human beings and guinea pigs after vaccination with the tick vaccine for spotted fever.

10.10 The Erythrocyte-Sensitizing Substances (ESS)

When suspensions of rickettsiae grown in the yolk-sac membrane are extracted with ether, the rickettsiae and soluble antigen are found in the aqueous phase. If sodium hydroxide is then added and the mixture is heated for thirty minutes at 100° C, the resultant material can be dialyzed against an isotonic phosphate buffer, and the erythrocyte-sensitizing substance (ESS) will remain in the dialysis bag (101). This substance is titrated by determining the least amount necessary to sensitize completely a certain volume of washed human erythrocytes under standard conditions.

Tests with immune sera indicate that the ESS from Rocky Mountain spotted fever, rickettsialpox, boutonneuse fever, and South African tick bite fever are probably common and group-specific.

The ESS test compares favorably with the complement-fixation and Weil-Felix tests in the early detection of antibodies. It is more sensitive and technically simpler than the C-F test, and is superior to the Weil-Felix reaction in that it has been positive in all cases of Rocky Mountain spotted fever or rickettsialpox. It appears to be a useful laboratory method for the diagnosis of the Rocky Mountain spotted fever group. Unfortunately, however, this reaction is not observed in experimental animals.

10.11 The Hemagglutination Method

Mel'nikov (102) found that antigenic substances such as polysaccharide haptenes are absorbed by rat erythrocytes, which can then be agglutinated by the corresponding immune sera. On the basis of this principle he devised a hemagglutination test, which is both sensitive and specific for rickettsial diseases belonging to the typhus and tick-borne spotted fever group. Mel'nikov recommended it as a new serologic method of diagnosis for these diseases.

10.12 The Fluorescent Antibody Technique

The fluorescent antibody technique originated by Coons in 1950 is so sensitive that the rickettsiae of epidemic typhus were identified by this method in a single infected human body louse (103). It was ten years before this technique was evaluated further for the visualization of pathogens in arthropod vectors. In 1960, Burgdorfer and Lackman (104) used antibodies labeled with fluorescein isothiocyanate to determine infection rates among *Dermacentor andersoni* fed on guinea pigs infected with *Rickettsia rickettsii*. In smears of gut tissues from infected nymphal ticks, the organisms stained consistently with a very bright fluorescence; in those prepared from adult ticks several weeks after molting, the rickettsiae, although still detectable, showed only a weak fluorescence.

10.13 Mechanism of "Reactivation"

The finding of noninfectious antigens in infected ticks was reported by Shepard and Goldwasser (105) in 1960.

The phenomenon of "reactivation," previously reported by Parker (85), is explained on the basis of this non-infectious antigen. When ticks containing this antigen, but no infectious rickettsiae, are allowed to feed on guinea pigs, the result is immunization of the guinea pigs without infection. Once the ticks have been fed or incubated, the rickettsiae are converted to a phase capable of multiplication in guinea pigs.

10.14 Detection of Antigen Early in the Clinical Disease

It has already been stated that none of the laboratory procedures currently in use can reliably make the diagnosis of Rocky Mountain spotted fever during the first week of the illness.

Theoretically, at least, rickettsial antigen in small concentrations should be present in the tissues and extracellular fluids of the host as soon as rickettsial infection occurs. A sensitive and specific method for detecting this antigen would be most useful in the early diagnosis of such infections. In 1947 Fleck (106) actually recovered such a specific soluble antigen from the urine of patients with typhus fever as early as the second day after onset. This antigen formed a precipitate with serum containing antibodies to typhus or to *Proteus X-19*. In rabbits inoculated with this soluble substance, a Weil-Felix antibody titer of 1:160 developed. A vaccine prepared from the urine of patients with typhus fever was actually used in an unsuccessful attempt to induce immunity to epidemic typhus.

Russian investigators (107, 108) have reported the detection of an antigen in the serum of patients with typhus fever during the first few days of fever. Of 107 patients studied during the preeruptive stage of typhus fever, approximately 60 per cent had this specific substance in their blood in amounts sufficient to be detected by complement-fixation. The circulating antigen was no longer demonstrable after specific antibodies appeared between the sixth and the ninth day of fever.

Attempts made several years ago (109) to demonstrate such a specific antigen in the urine of patients with Rocky Mountain spotted fever were unsuccessful. No recent studies on this promising lead have been reported.

CHAPTER XI

Pathophysiology

11.1 Neglect of Studies on Pathologic Physiology

The histologic hallmark of Rocky Mountain spotted fever, first described by Wolbach (32) in 1919, is the intranuclear localization of the rickettsiae in the vascular endothelium and in the smooth-muscle cells of the walls of blood vessels. This knowledge was not correlated with the clinical picture until the 1940s, most of the effort in the intervening period being devoted to studies of the ecology, etiology, and immunology of spotted fever. The treatment of the individual was confined to "general supportive measures and the relief of symptoms" (110). The administration of intravenous fluids or blood was actually interdicted, apparently because of poor past experience with patients so treated (111, 112).

11.2 Correlation of Pathologic Anatomy with Pathologic Physiology

The careful clinical studies first reported in 1944 by Harrell, Venning, and Wolff (110) revealed the pathologic physiology of Rocky Mountain spotted fever and explained why properly selected intravenous supportive therapy is so beneficial.

Early in the course of spotted fever, the patient may have a moderate amount of generalized edema involving the face, eyes, hands, and legs. This edema is firm in consistency and does not tend to localize in the dependent portions of the body. The explanation offered by Harrell (113) was that capillary permeability is increased in spotted fever, just as it is in severe burns. In spotted fever the capillary change is due to direct injury by the rickettsiae, whereas in burns it is due to "toxins." The increased capillary permeability causes a leakage of plasma proteins—albumin in particular—into the interstitial fluid space, thus decreasing intravascular osmotic pressure. The plasma volume is decreased during the peak period of the disease and returns to normal during convalescence (114). Early in the disease, the circulating red-cell volume may be unchanged; the disproportionate loss of plasma causes hemoconcentration, and the hematocrit increases. With the development of the rash, a visible manifestation of the extravasation of erythrocytes into the tissues, both the circulating red-cell volume and the hematocrit are decreased.

The presence of serum proteins in the interstitial fluid explains the nonpitting generalized edema found clinically. Evidences for expansion of the extracellular fluid space are an increase in the thiocyanate space (114), clinical edema, and an increase in body weight. The intravenous infusion of crystalloids alone aggravates the clinical edema. Only when crystalloid therapy is preceded by the infusion of plasma and whole blood to increase the intravascular osmotic pressure and to bolster the plasma volume is parenteral therapy successful.

11.3 Consequences of Dehydration

In patients severely ill with spotted fever, the oral intake of both fluids and food may be inadequate (113). The fluid loss resulting from perspiration and fever is often aggravated by salicylate therapy. In many cases prerenal azotemia develops, the blood nonprotein nitrogen rising to levels of 70 to 90 mg per 100 ml. At the same time, the serum chloride concentration may decrease to a range of 75 to 85 mEq per liter. Ordinarily, such deficits of water and crystalloids would call for replacement therapy consisting in the intravenous infusion of glucose (a 5 per cent solution in water) and sodium chloride solution (0.85 per cent).

In the first patient studied by Harrell and his co-workers, the administration of these agents promptly corrected the abnormal chemical values, but the patient's clinical condition became worse: the edema increased, and the blood pressure dropped to shock levels. It was then recognized that the circulating blood volume was not being maintained and that the hypoproteinemia had worsened. When the administration of crystalloids was preceded by plasma or whole blood given parenterally to increase the intravascular osmotic pressure, the patients improved.

Tremendous amounts of protein or whole blood may be needed. A two-year-old child weighing 11.7 Kg received a total of 2,800 cc of fluids in a period of ten days, and a fifteen-year-old boy was given 2,500 cc of plasma in thirty-six hours. Purified human serum albumin was very effective, although expensive.

11.4 Disorders of Protein Metabolism

Definite histopathologic evidence of hepatic damage is seen at autopsy in fatal cases of spotted fever. The clinical signs of liver involvement are icterus, decreased excretion of hippuric acid, and hypoalbuminemia. The degree of functional hepatic impairment appears to parallel closely the clinical severity of the disease. Serial studies show that this impairment may persist well into the fifth week, but that liver function returns to normal during convalescence. Determinations of urinary nitrogen output in a fifteen-year-old male patient (115) revealed that the equivalent of 561 gm of dry protein or seven pounds of skeletal muscle was excreted in seventy-eight hours. The hypoproteinemia results from nitrogen breakdown (which is associated with the infection and fever), together with the decreased oral intake of food, the presumably decreased hepatic synthesis of protein, and the sequestration of plasma proteins in the interstitial fluid space.

11.5 Results of Protein Replacement

In a group of patients with Rocky Mountain spotted fever, Harrell and his associates (116) tried the effect of a high oral intake of protein (3 to 4 gm per kilogram of body weight). In comparison with a control group, the patients receiving the high-protein diet appeared to have fewer toxic symptoms, fewer neurologic manifestations, less necrosis of the skin, and less edema. Almost without exception, the patients gained weight during the course of their illness. Although the degree of clinical improvement was more striking than the increase in the concentration of the blood proteins, the amount of intravenous albumin, plasma, or blood required to support the circulation was less than in the control group.

11.6 Peripheral Circulatory Collapse

Spotted fever is associated with one of the most severe forms of peripheral circulatory collapse, which usually develops in the second week of rash. The clinical picture—

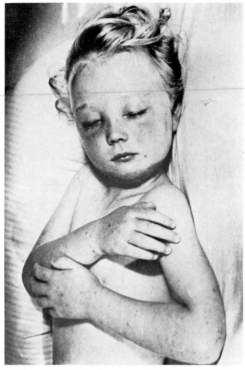

FIGURE 7. Edema in a four-and-one-half-year-old girl treated with
supportive therapy alone.
1. Eighth day of rash. Pronounced edema has led to partial
closure of the eyes and puffiness of the hands.

tachycardia, hypotension, depression of the sensorium,
and pallor—is associated with a decrease in plasma volume
and, usually, with hypoproteinemia. This "toxic" condition is strikingly similar to early "shock" associated with
functional capillary damage from any cause. Experimentally, such a picture of shock may be produced by
burns, bacterial toxins, or other substances. If treated
early enough, the changes are reversible. The intravenous

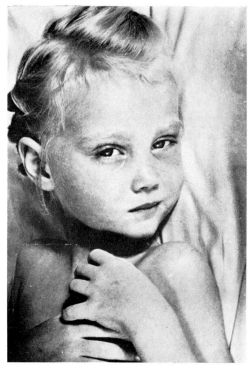

2. One month after onset. With recovery, the edema has
disappeared.

administration of plasma and whole blood is the treatment
of choice.

The peripheral circulatory collapse seen in spotted fever
also resembles the shock resulting from adrenal cortical
failure which is seen in cases of meningococcemia and
acute adrenal insufficiency. It is possible that the blood
supply to the adrenal cortex is compromised by the
vascular lesions of spotted fever. The value of adrenal
cortical hormones in alleviating the symptoms of toxicity
in spotted fever is discussed in Chapter 13.

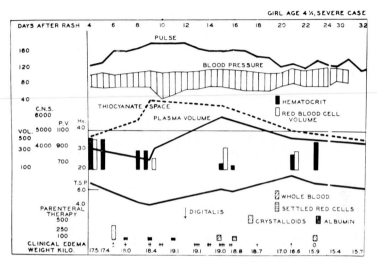

FIGURE 8. The pathophysiology of severe Rocky Mountain spotted fever in the girl shown in Figures 7.1 and 7.2, who was treated with supportive therapy alone.

Note the gradual rise in pulse rate and increase in thiocyanate space (C.N.S.), accompanied by a fall in the diastolic blood pressure, plasma volume (P.V.), and total serum protein content (T.S.P.). With the administration of serum albumin, the plasma volume rose 6 cc for every gm of albumin injected. The increase in plasma volume and the return of capillary integrity were followed by the development of central (myocardial) circulatory failure, requiring the administration of digitalis.

11.7 Reproduction of the Physiologic Changes of Spotted Fever During Serum Sickness

The administration of antiserum to a three-year-old girl with moderately severe spotted fever decreased the toxic symptoms but did not prevent the alterations in capillary permeability (114). As the thiocyanate space increased, the plasma volume and the serum protein content dropped, and edema developed. With the restoration of capillary integrity during clinical recovery (manifested by a drop in temperature and a decrease in toxic symptoms), the edema disappeared and the thiocyanate space decreased, although the plasma volume remained low. When serum sickness developed, the patient again became edematous and the thiocyanate space increased markedly; the plasma volume and serum protein content, however, showed little change.

The similarity of the changes observed during serum sickness to those observed during the course of spotted fever suggested the operation of an immune mechanism in the alteration of capillary permeability.

11.8 Similarity of Serum Sickness to Rocky Mountain Spotted Fever

Serum sickness was produced in rabbits by the administration of human plasma. The initial appearance of humoral antibody was associated with an increase in the thiocyanate space, a decrease in plasma volume and in serum protein, and the development of cutaneous edema. It appeared that an in-vivo antigen-antibody reaction had increased capillary permeability (117), producing changes which resembled those observed experimentally in rabbits infected with Rocky Mountain spotted fever (118, 119). In a later series of experiments (120), rabbits sensitized with human plasma also showed an increased radiosodium space in the adrenal glands (120). Although the exact significance of this latter finding is not clear, it suggests an association between adrenal cortical function and immune mechanisms, and lends weight to the theory that severe adrenal cortical dysfunction may contribute to the shock observed clinically in spotted fever.

11.9 Pathogenesis of Central (Myocardial) Circulatory Failure

In some of Harrell's cases, myocardial failure as well as peripheral circulatory collapse was observed in patients with spotted fever (114); in others, congestive heart failure was precipitated by therapy. Not all his patients showed changes in the electrocardiogram, and few electro-cardiographic readings were made during the acute episodes of congestive failure. The changes that were observed were similar to those seen in beriberi, myxedema, and anasarca from other causes.

In fatal cases of Rocky Mountain spotted fever, sections of the myocardium usually show edema of the muscle fibers; in some cases, lesions resembling periarteritis nodosa have been seen in small blood vessels. Two mechanisms may be involved in the myocardial failure: (1) the mechanical interference produced by edema, and (2) anoxia resulting from the involvement of arterioles.

In one reported case of spotted fever intermittent nodal tachycardia, discovered during the course of the illness, persisted after clinical recovery (121).

11.10 Thrombocytopenia and Hypofibrinogenemia

That thrombocytopenia may accompany spotted fever was not recognized until 1960, when Phillips and his associates (122) found a platelet count of 21,550 per cubic millimeter in a patient with the disease. In 1963, Mengel and Trygstad (123) reported a count of 6,000 per cubic millimeter in a patient who died.

A case of spotted fever with severe hypofibrinogenemia as well as thrombocytopenia has been reported recently (124). The platelet count was 12,000 per cubic milli-meter, and the plasma fibrinogen level was 4 mg per

100 ml; the patient's blood failed to clot in a test tube. After treatment with antibiotics, methylprednisolone, human fibrinogen, blood, and plasma, the patient recovered. The development of the hypofibrinogenemia was explained on the basis of the diffuse vasculitis, which set the stage for the entry of thromboplastin and plasminogen activator into the circulation, for defibrination due to multiple vascular thromboses, for accelerated intravascular clotting and fibrinolysis, and for hepatic damage leading to reduced production of clotting factors by the liver.

11.11 Neurologic Changes

Involvement of the central nervous system during acute spotted fever may be manifested clinically by confusion, coma, convulsions, hyperactive and pathologic reflexes, cranial nerve palsies, paraplegia, and hemiplegia. These neurologic changes may persist for weeks or months after the onset of the illness. They usually subside without residual signs or symptoms, but permanent sequelae remain in some cases (125-127). Thirty-seven of Harrell's patients who had recovered from spotted fever were re-examined one to eight years later for evidences of residual neurologic damage (126). The history, physical examination, or electroencephalogram revealed some type of neurologic sequelae in twenty-one of the thirty-seven patients. Fourteen gave a history of symptoms related to the central nervous system; six had neurologic signs; and twelve had clearly abnormal electroencephalograms.

In six of Harrell's patients who died during the acute illness and whose brains were examined at necropsy, microinfarcts or granulomas were found adjacent to cerebral blood vessels.

CHAPTER XII

Prevention

12.1 Avoidance of Infection

Man is an accidental host of the tick vector of Rocky Mountain spotted fever. The most certain way to avoid infection would be to stay out of areas where ticks are numerous. While it may be feasible for most persons to observe this precaution in certain localities in the Rocky Mountain states, it would not be so in the East or South, where dog ticks are the vectors.

12.2 Individual Prophylaxis

The most effective form of individual prophylaxis against spotted fever lies in preventing the attachment of a tick to the skin, or removing it as quickly as possible if it becomes attached. Since victims are seldom aware of crawling ticks, or even of the process of attachment, frequent inspection of the scalp, skin, and clothing is necessary in tick-infested areas (128).

As a rule, the head of an attached tick is embedded beneath the surface of the skin, while the body remains free and protrudes at an angle. A tick which has attached itself recently can often be removed by gentle traction applied to its body. If inspection of the tick upon removal reveals the head to be missing, it must be removed separately. The piece of skin in which the head lies embedded may be snipped off with a fine pair of scissors after being elevated with a pair of forceps, or the point of a hypodermic needle or scalpel may be used to remove the head.

In removing a tick, one should be extremely careful not to crush it. Engorged ticks must be removed with forceps or gauze-protected fingers. If an engorged tick is accidentally crushed, the discharged contents should be thoroughly washed from the skin with soap and water, care being taken not to irritate the skin.

12.3 Methods of Tick Control

Once ticks have taken up their abode in populated areas, eradication is most difficult, and may take months or years. DDT in solution or incorporated in an aerosol insecticide may be effective. A powder containing DDT (10 per cent) destroys ticks which infest small pets. It can be applied liberally and is not dangerous to animals.

In suburban areas, roadside and pathside control of *Dermacentor variabilis* and *Amblyomma americanum* is easily attained with insecticides (129). Such methods of control have a very definite application in inhabited areas where the incidence of spotted fever is high, or even where ticks are annoyingly plentiful. Dusts, sprays, mists, and possibly even fogs made with DDT (2.5 lbs. of actual insecticide per acre) or chlordane (1 lb. per acre) are reasonably effective. It is conceivable that some of the newer insecticides, such as dieldrin, will prove even more useful.

12.4 Vaccination

Thanks to Howard Ricketts and the other scientists whose efforts to develop a vaccine have been described in Chapter VII, Rocky Mountain spotted fever is now preventable. Complete protection is afforded by annual vaccination with either the chick-embryo vaccine or the tick vaccine. The dose of the chick-embryo vaccine, now commercially available in ample amounts, is 0.5 cc for children under twelve years of age and 1 cc for older children and adults. The vaccine is injected subcutaneously. For the initial course of immunization, three doses at intervals of a week or ten days are recommended. Booster doses are needed each year. Although one such injection is deemed adequate, it is customary to give two doses a week or ten days apart.

In the Rocky Mountain areas the vaccine should be given very early in the spring, since wood ticks begin to feed as soon as snow leaves the ground. In other sections of the country, the vaccine may be administered later in the spring. The development of peak immunity requires four to six weeks.

Persons who are allergic to eggs or chickens may react unfavorably to the chick-embryo vaccine. For such patients, the tick vaccine is still available.

Exposure to Rocky Mountain spotted fever is not general enough to warrant a mass vaccination program, except occasionally in certain areas where the disease is unusually prevalent. The vaccine should be given, however, to all whose business or pleasure takes them into localities where ticks are encountered in appreciable numbers or from which cases of the diseases have been reported in the recent past.

CHAPTER XIII

Treatment

13.1 Support of the Patient

Once a diagnosis of spotted fever has been made, therapy should be considered in two parts: (1) support of the patient, and (2) antirickettsial measures. Prior to the early 1940s, the management of Rocky Mountain spotted fever consisted solely in general supportive therapy, which included good nursing care and diet and the treatment of complicating diseases or conditions. In 1944 the importance of attention to the pathologic physiology of the disease was recognized by Harrell, Venning, and Wolff (110). The newer concepts of supportive treatment, introduced by Harrell and his associates, have been discussed in Chapter XI.

13.2 Treatment with Immune Sera

In 1908, Ricketts (16) found that the blood of a guinea pig which had recovered from Rocky Mountain spotted fever had a specific protective effect when it was injected, with a few rickettsiae, into normal guinea pigs. He later demonstrated a specific antibody in the sera of rabbits and horses that had been inoculated with the spotted fever organism. With sera from these animals Ricketts conferred a short-lived passive immunity upon guinea pigs. He subsequently immunized two guinea pigs with a combination of rickettsiae and immune serum, and demonstrated that the immunity lasted at least sixty-seven days. Noguchi (43) subsequently repeated this work, and in one animal secured immunity that lasted at least thirteen months. His unsuccessful attempt to immunize human subjects with this material has been mentioned in Chapter VII. Other attempts at *serotherapy* in human beings were in general unsatisfactory until 1943.

In 1940, Topping (130) developed an immune rabbit serum of high potency. When 5 cc of this serum was administered subcutaneously to infected guinea pigs during the first two days of fever, the disease was of shorter duration than in untreated infected guinea pigs used as controls; furthermore, all of the control animals died, while all those treated survived. This immune rabbit serum was next concentrated twenty-fold (131). In guinea pigs the therapeutic effect of the concentrated serum (1 ml per kilogram of body weight) varied inversely with the time elapsing between inoculation with rickettsiae and administration of the serum. During the summers of 1941 and 1942, this immune rabbit serum was administered to seventy-one human patients with spotted fever. Nineteen were treated after the third day of rash (on the sixth or seventh day of illness), and they received little, if any, benefit. Of the fifty-two patients treated before the third day of rash only two died, and these were elderly (66 and 72 years old). The fatality rate in the treated group (3.8 per cent) was far lower than the expected rate of 19 per cent.

The rickettsiae of Rocky Mountain spotted fever are at first intracellular but become intranuclear as the disease progresses. The antibody contained in immune serum, a gamma globulin, is too large a molecule readily to penetrate the living cell. Immune serum, therefore, can be

effective only in the early stages of spotted fever before
rickettsiae in large numbers have become established in
the cellular nuclei.

13.3 Chemotherapy

Chemotherapy with sulfonamides, so dramatically effective against certain bacteria, proved of no value against
the rickettsiae in experimental animals (130); these drugs,
in fact, had a deleterious effect (132). Fitzpatrick (133)
reported that sulfapyridine and sulfathiazole were con-
traindicated in spotted fever, since deaths occurred earlier
in guinea pigs treated with these drugs than in the
controls.

13.4 Para-aminobenzoic Acid (PABA) as an Antirickettsial Agent

At the outbreak of the second World War, the expecta-
tion that typhus fever and other rickettsial diseases would
become military problems stimulated intensive investigations of chemotherapeutic agents that might be effective
against rickettsiae. Snyder, Maier, and Anderson (134),
after finding that the sulfonamides enhance the multiplication of rickettsiae in infected animals, hypothesized
that the antagonism noted between the sulfonamides and
para-aminobenzoic acid (PABA) in bacterial infections
might work in reverse in rickettsial infections. Greiff,
Pinkerton, and Moragues (135), working independently,
found that PABA appeared to enhance the action of
penicillin. Studying PABA further, they used the
rickettsiae of murine typhus, cultivated on yolk sacs of
developing eggs, to establish the rickettsiostatic effect of
PABA. All mice infected with this agent and fed PABA
orally survived, whereas all of the control animals died.

In 1943 and 1944, an epidemic of louse-borne typhus in Cairo, Egypt, provided the opportunity for a clinical trial of PABA. In patients treated with the drug (2 gm given orally every two hours in 25 cc of a 5 per cent solution of sodium bicarbonate), the blood level of free PABA was kept between 10 and 20 mg per 100 cc. Treatment was continued until the body temperature returned to normal, the average amount of PABA received by each patient being 127 gm. No deaths occurred among the seventeen patients so treated, whereas the mortality among forty-four untreated patients was 18 per cent. The clinical severity of the disease, as well as the duration of fever, was considerably lessened in the treated group (136).

These significant observations on the activity of PABA in typhus fever led Anigstein and Bader (137), as well as Hamilton (138), to extend the investigation to experimental Rocky Mountain spotted fever. PABA was shown to arrest the multiplication of *R. rickettsii* in embryonated eggs and in guinea pigs. This inhibitory effect on the rickettsiae was more striking in spotted fever than in typhus.

13.5 Clinical Treatment of Spotted Fever with PABA

Rose, Duane, and Fischel (139) were the first investigators to report a human case of spotted fever treated with PABA. In their patient, clinical improvement began within twenty-four hours after PABA was started; the fever declined continuously thereafter, and recovery was rapid and uneventful. Many other reports of similar favorable results soon followed (140-142).

Woodward and Raby (143) reported seventeen cases of spotted fever treated with PABA without a fatality.

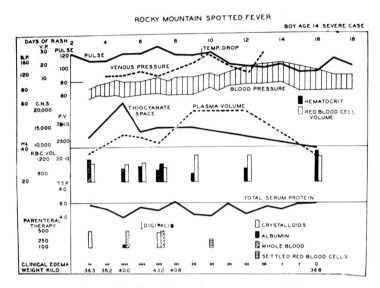

FIGURE 9. The pathophysiology of severe spotted fever in a boy aged fourteen, treated with antiserum and para-aminobenzoic acid.

The patient was severely ill on admission to the hospital. The pulse rate and the thiocyanate space were increased and the blood pressure was low; the plasma volume and the serum protein content were not altered. With hydration, an increase in the thiocyanate space and a fall in the serum protein content occurred simultaneously with the development of notable clinical edema. Antiserum was administered daily from the third to the sixth day of rash, with little improvement. Administration of para-aminobenzoic acid (PABA) was then started, the peak blood levels being attained between the ninth and eleventh days of rash, when clinical recovery usually begins. Central circulatory failure, which developed with the rise in plasma volume, was controlled with digitalis. As convalescence progressed, the blood pressure rose, the pulse rate decreased, and the plasma volume, thiocyanate space, and serum protein content returned to normal. A high oral intake of PABA (approximately 5 gm per kgm of body weight daily) was maintained. Antihistaminic drugs were administered, but not until the twenty-second day of rash, after the circulatory changes had reverted to normal.   ⫸⟶

In this series the average duration of the entire febrile course was 6.8 days; the average duration of fever after drug administration, 3.0 days; and the average period of hospitalization, 11.9 days. All three of these figures are less than the comparable averages for cases of spotted fever not treated with PABA.

Although PABA was of definite value in the treatment of spotted fever, it was not the ideal drug. Large doses, almost to the limit of tolerance, had to be given every two hours, and the drug was of little value unless given relatively early in the disease. Because of its toxicity, many laboratory procedures were required to supervise its administration adequately. It occasionally produced leukopenia, and many patients treated with PABA showed 3- to 4-plus cephalin flocculation reactions and significant reductions in prothrombin time. Finally, although the over-all results were statistically significant, the immediate clinical improvement in the patient's condition was not dramatic.

13.6 The Mode of Action of PABA

It has been shown in chick embryos that rickettsiae grow rapidly in slowly growing or dying cells (138). In contrast, their growth is greatly impeded when cells are rapidly metabolizing, as in mice fed methylene blue or toluidine blue (144) or in chick eggs incubated at temperatures higher than 37° C. In addition to its rickettsiostatic action, PABA increases the oxygen con-

---

The necessity for meticulous attention to every minor detail of supportive therapy is well illustrated by this case; it was the unanimous opinion of all the physicians up to the tenth day of rash that the patient would die.

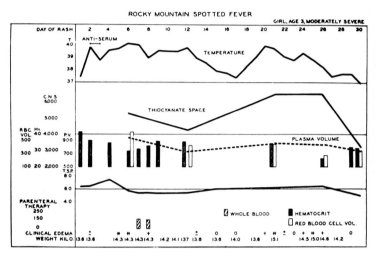

FIGURE 10. The pathophysiology of moderately severe spotted fever and of serum sickness in a patient treated with antiserum.

The patient showed signs of dehydration and toxemia on admission to the hospital. The administration of antiserum decreased the toxic symptoms but did not prevent the alterations in capillary permeability. As the thiocyanate space increased, the plasma volume and serum protein content dropped, and edema developed. With the restoration of capillary integrity during clinical recovery (manifested by the fall in temperature and the lessening of toxic symptoms), the edema disappeared and the thiocyanate space decreased, but the plasma volume remained low. When serum sickness developed, edema returned and the thiocyanate space increased markedly, although the plasma volume and serum protein content showed little change. Benadryl® was given. After the patient recovered from serum sickness and the edema disappeared, the thiocyanate space, plasma volume, and serum protein content all decreased.

sumption of both normal and infected chick embryos. The meta and ortho compounds of aminobenzoic acid, on the other hand, are not rickettsiostatic and have no effect on oxygen consumption. Such a high degree of specificity suggests that PABA may act on an enzyme system. The finding of rickettsiostasis with increased oxygen consumption seems to be the counterpart of the observation that sublethal amounts of potassium cyanide, which decreases metabolism and oxygen consumption, favor the growth of rickettsiae under certain conditions (145). Cyanide, however, has no effect on the rickettsiostatic action of PABA. Greiff (146) concluded that PABA either acts directly on the rickettsiae, in a manner similar to the action of sulfonamides on some bacteria, or, like toluidine blue, increases cell respiration by short-circuiting the cyanide-sensitive system of respiratory enzymes.

Since PABA possesses only rickettsiostatic properties, the infection must be overcome by the immune mechanisms of the host. The drug serves merely to arrest the growth and development of invading rickettsiae while these mechanisms become operative. PABA has no effect on rickettsiae already in the body, nor does it repair damage already done by the disease.

13.7 Antibiotics

In 1946, reasonably satisfactory methods for the diagnosis and prevention of Rocky Mountain spotted fever were available, while treatment of the disease was still far from adequate. With the discovery of antibiotics— chemicals obtained from soil bacteria and molds—hope was raised that some of these agents would possess rickettsiostatic ability. Penicillin was even more successful than the sulfonamides in the treatment of some bacterial diseases, but was ineffective against rickettsiae. Streptomycin also proved ineffective. The discovery of Aureomycin, however, opened a new chapter in the control of rickettsial diseases.

13.8 Aureomycin (Chlortetracycline)

Aureomycin, so named because of the golden color of colonies of the mold, was isolated from *Streptomyces auriofaciens* by Duggar (147) in 1948, after he had screened 3,400 strains of fungus-like organisms or molds. Subsequent studies on the chemical structure of Aureomycin have identified it as the 7-chloroderivative of tetracycline. Wong and Cox (148) found that Aureomycin protected guinea pigs and mice infected with typhus, Rocky Mountain spotted fever, Q fever, and rickettsialpox.

In June, 1948, Ross and his coworkers (149) began using Aureomycin for the treatment of spotted fever. They reported that in thirteen patients treated with daily doses of 60 mg per kilogram of body weight the blood level of the drug ranged from 0.3 to 2.5 micrograms per milliliter. The only toxic manifestations were occasional transient nausea and vomiting, which did not contraindicate the continuation of therapy. The results obtained in these thirteen patients were compared with those obtained in thirty cases treated supportively and symptomatically between 1932 and 1945, and in seventeen patients treated with PABA in 1946 and 1947.

In the group given supportive treatment only, the mortality rate was 10 per cent. The mean duration of fever was 18 days; rash persisted for twelve days, usually becoming petechial after the first week. The mean hospital stay was twenty days, and complications (including pneumonia, myocarditis, and parotitis) occurred in 27 per cent of the cases. There were no deaths among the seventeen patients treated with para-aminobenzoic acid. The mean duration of fever following initiation of PABA therapy was six days, and the rash generally persisted for six days. The mean duration of hospitalization was twelve days. Eighteen per cent of the patients had complications. In the thirteen patients treated with Aureomycin during the summer of 1948, the temperature response was more dramatic, the average duration of fever after the beginning of Aureomycin therapy being two and one-third days. The mean duration of the rash was four days. The average hospital stay was eight days, and there were no complications.

Aureomycin is readily absorbed after oral administration. When single doses are given, appreciable amounts may be recovered from the urine within short periods of time. Maximum urinary concentrations occur within two to eight hours, although excretion of Aureomycin may continue for as long as two or three days. Satisfactory blood levels seem to be established within four to six hours after an oral dose, and are apparently maintained by additional doses of Aureomycin at intervals of six hours. The recommended daily dose is 50 to 100 mg per kilogram of body weight, divided into four equal doses. The rickettsiostatic action of chlortetracycline is probably accounted for by its diffusion into the intracellular water.

13.9 Chloromycetin (Chloramphenicol)

A sample of field soil from Venezuela yielded a mold of the genus *Actinomyces,* which was identified as a new species, *Streptomyces venezuelae.* From a broth culture of this new mold, Ehrlich and his coworkers (150) prepared a crystalline substance which was given the name *Chloromycetin* in recognition of its source and of the high content of nonionic chlorine that characterizes its molecule. It was synthesized in 1949 and given the chemical name *chloramphenicol.* Chloramphenicol is D-threo-(-)-1-p-nitrophenyl-2-dichloro-acetamido-1, 3-

propanediol. It is the first naturally occurring compound found to possess -NO_2 or -$COCHCl_2$ groups. The initial studies of its antibiotic spectrum, in vitro and in vivo in animals, indicated outstanding effectiveness in rickettsial infections of chick embryos and mice (151, 152).

Chloramphenicol was first administered to patients with Rocky Mountain spotted fever by Pincoffs and his associates (153) in 1948. They treated fifteen cases of the Eastern type with Chloromycetin, the initial dose of 50 to 75 mg per kilogram of body weight being followed by 0.25 to 0.5 gm every three hours. Improvement was not striking in the first twenty-four hours, but the eruption did not spread following the initiation of treatment and had markedly regressed by the end of the second day. Symptoms such as headache and mental dullness abated on the second day of treatment. On the third day, in the majority of cases, the patients were plainly convalescent. In all cases the temperature fell to normal within seventy-six hours, the average duration of fever after the initiation of therapy being 2.2 days. Blood studies showed a rapid disappearance of rickettsemia after therapy was begun, followed by the development of immune bodies as in the usual course of the disease.

The precise mechanism responsible for the effectiveness of chloramphenicol is still unknown. Because of the structural similarity between chloramphenicol and phenylalanine, it has been suggested that the drug inhibits the incorporation of this essential amino acid into protein, thereby interrupting rickettsial growth. Even in concentrations ten times as high as those usually obtained in the blood of patients, chloramphenicol is incapable of inactivating rickettsiae in vitro; hence it appears probable that it acts in vivo by inhibiting rather than killing rickettsiae. The drug does not have an antitoxic effect (154). Its sole beneficial action, like that of PABA, appears to be to suppress the growth of rickettsiae until the body has time to marshal its defenses. Patients treated with chloramphenicol may continue to harbor *R. rickettsii* for some time after recovery (155). Viable rickettsiae were isolated from the lymphatic tissue of a patient one year following recovery from Rocky Mountain spotted fever.

Chloramphenicol is administered orally. Although the drug is relatively insoluble in water, it is well absorbed from the gastrointestinal tract. After single doses, appreciable amounts can be demonstrated in both blood and urine within half an hour, the titers decreasing to zero at the end of eight hours. This drug is most effective against Rocky Mountain spotted fever when given early in the course of the disease. Since it does not repair damage that has already been done by the rickettsiae, early diagnosis is important. Therapy should be continued until the patient's temperature has been normal for forty-eight to seventy-two hours. Patients with spotted fever usually become afebrile within forty-eight to seventy-two hours after the initiation of chloramphenicol therapy; therefore the drug can be discontinued in most cases after four to six days. If a relapse occurs, another course of the antibiotic can be given, since there is no evidence that rickettsiae develop drug resistance.

The greatest disadvantage of chloramphenicol is that it sometimes causes fatal depression of hematopoiesis. Aplastic anemia may develop suddenly in patients who had previously tolerated the drug.

13.10 The Tetracyclines

At the present time, the drugs of choice in the treatment

of Rocky Mountain spotted fever are the tetracyclines. *Tetracycline* (Achromycin®, Panmycin®, Polycycline®, Tetracyn®), the parent compound, is a derivative of napthacenecarboxamide. It is a yellowish, odorless powder which is only slightly soluble in water. It is used in the form of the free base and as the hydrochloride, which is water-soluble. Tetracycline has the same general activity, uses, and side effects as oxytetracycline and chlortetracycline, and is used in the same doses.

Chlortetracycline (Aureomycin) has already been mentioned. *Oxytetracycline* (Terramycin), a bright yellow ampholyte readily soluble in water, is derived from the soil actinomycete, *Streptomyces rimosus*. It is relatively nontoxic. It is the 5-hydroxy derivative of tetracycline, and it closely resembles chlortetracycline in its action. In the original report on oxytetracycline by Finlay and his associates (156), antirickettsial effects in the chick embryo were described. Subsequent experimental and clinical studies substantiated this antirickettsial action (157).

The first two cases of Rocky Mountain spotted fever treated with Terramycin were in children, aged three and four years, who began receiving Terramycin orally on the fourth and tenth days of the disease. Initial doses of 1 and 0.75 gm were followed by doses of 250 to 500 mg given every eight hours until the temperature reached normal. The headache and other signs of toxicity improved dramatically within twenty-four hours, and the temperature returned permanently to normal levels in sixty and forty-eight hours. Convalescence was entirely uneventful in both cases. The blood levels of Terramycin ranged from 1.2 to 11 micrograms per cubic centimeter, the mean level being 4.4 micrograms per cubic centimeter.

Following a single dose of 2 gm (in adults), appreciable concentrations of Terramycin may be detected in the blood for twenty-four hours. The subsequent administration of 0.5 gm every six hours will maintain a therapeutic blood level. The drug penetrates the cells and is found in the body fluids, including the spinal fluid. The most serious side-effect of oxytetracycline is intestinal irritation. In some patients it causes anorexia, nausea, vomiting, and persistent diarrhea sometimes leading to proctitis.

13.11 Mechanism of the Rickettsiostatic Action of Antibiotics

The tetracyclines in high concentrations inhibit the synthesis of protein in bacteria, and uncouple oxidative phosphorylation in liver and kidney homogenates. Both thyroxin and tetracycline appear to effect uncoupling by interaction with the magnesium ion. *In vitro,* these substances produce uncoupling only when the drugs are incubated in a medium low in magnesium content. The addition of an excess of magnesium will prevent or reverse the inhibition of phosphorylation.

It is probable that the inhibitory effect of chlortetracycline, oxytetracycline, and chloramphenicol on rickettsiae may be due to the removal of the magnesium ion from the reaction medium (158).

A recent study (159), however, suggests that uncoupling agents operate by interfering with the synthesis of high-energy intermediates, and not by hydrolyzing or otherwise inactivating them.

In vivo, tetracycline and chlortetracycline are adsorbed immediately to bone and, once deposited, are retained for long intervals (160). All three of the antibiotics under discussion—chlortetracycline, oxytetracycline, and chloramphenicol—combine specifically with the mitochondria of living cells, both in tissue cultures and in fresh preparations from various organs (161). As this combination occurs, oxidative phosphorylation is decreased in the mitochondria.

It is apparent that the biochemical, enzymatic, and intracellular mechanisms of rickettsial infections and of antibiotic action require further study. At the present, the most likely explanation for the rickettsiostatic action of these drugs appears to be that they bind magnesium ion in the mitochondria and in nuclei, thereby inhibiting oxidative phosphorylation and the synthesis of protein.

13.12 The Use of Cortisone as an Adjunct

Therapy with the antibiotic agents usually does not bring the temperature to normal for a period of 2.5 to four days. In a severely ill patient the management of the toxemia, dehydration, hypochloremia, hypoproteinemia, and peripheral circulatory collapse so characteristic of late Rocky Mountain spotted fever may remain a difficult problem even after the initiation of antibiotic therapy.

It is of historic interest that Smith (162), in 1913, treated three cases of spotted fever with adrenaline (glandular extract) and reported a shortening of the course of the infection. In 1953, Aikawa and Harrell (163) reported experimental studies in guinea pigs infected with *R. rickettsii* and treated with cortisone acetate in doses comparable to those employed in human beings. These studies suggested that this hormone reduced the mortality rate in animals with moderately severe infections. The reported effectiveness of adrenal cortical hormones in ameliorating the toxemia of pneumonia and typhoid fever (164) prompted Arney (165) and Workman (166) to try cortisone combined with a specific antibiotic in the treatment of spotted fever.

In the latter study, nine unselected patients were given cortisone orally or intramuscularly in addition to chloramphenicol. Adults received an initial dose of 200 mg, followed by two doses of 100 mg each, at six-hour intervals. Children were given approximately two thirds of this dose. In no case did the total duration of cortisone therapy exceed twelve hours. Therapy was begun between the fourth and thirteenth days of the disease, the mean being 6.3 days. Clinical improvement was uniformly observed within twenty-four hours or less after the institution of the combined therapy. The most striking observations were alleviation of the headache and other toxic symptoms, and return of the patient's appetite. All patients survived. The mean duration of fever after the institution of treatment was 1.8 days, as compared with 3.3 days in thirty patients who received chloramphenicol alone, and 2.5 days in patients treated with Terramycin. Supplemental therapy with adrenocortical hormones thus appears to be of definite benefit in patients first treated late in the course of the disease. The exact mechanism of this salutary effect is not known, but the clinical similarity between severe Rocky Mountain spotted fever and adrenal insufficiency has already been pointed out.

13.13 Effect of Antibiotics and Cortisone on the Immune Reaction

Guinea pigs infected with spotted fever organisms and treated with Aureomycin were immune to reinoculation with homologous rickettsiae following their recovery; Aureomycin did not seem to interfere with the immune mechanism. Complement-fixing antibodies also appeared in the treated animals (167). When cortisone (25 mg daily for eight to twelve days) was injected into guinea pigs being immunized against spotted fever with the specific vaccine, the level of specific complement-fixing antibody was lowered slightly (167).

In patients treated with Chloromycetin (153), immune bodies developed as in the usual course of Rocky Mountain spotted fever. It is conceivable, however, that the initiation of antibiotic therapy early in the course of the disease would suppress antibody formation, and Flinn (168) has reported six cases, treated with chloramphenicol or tetracycline, in which the Weil-Felix and complement-fixation tests were negative. The possibility of a misdiagnosis must always be considered under such circumstances.

The availability of effective antibiotic agents has adversely affected the reporting of all rickettsial infections. So many cases are aborted by early treatment with such agents that diagnosis with complete laboratory confirmation is becoming a rarity. Since the development of complement-fixing antibodies might be delayed sometimes for six months or more, confirmation of diagnosis in recent years has been largely the result of epidemiologic follow-up of cases by public health agencies.

CHAPTER XIV

Summing Up

Many superstitions have some basis in common sense. The Shoshone braves were cowardly but clever, to expose only their squaws to the "evil spirits" associated with the gophers in the foothills of the Rockies. In avoiding areas inhabited by the evil spirits, the Indians practiced effective prophylaxis—the prevention of accidental exposure to the tick. This is still the best means of avoiding Rocky Mountain spotted fever.

The Indians were so attuned to their environment that they were a part of its natural ecology, and spotted fever was not to them a great health hazard. When the white settlers moved in, they brought along large domesticated hosts for the ticks in the form of cattle, sheep, and horses. As the tick population multiplied closer to established human habitations, Rocky Mountain spotted fever became a problem to human beings.

The pioneer physician may have been poorly trained by present standards, but he did possess the faculty for careful, detailed clinical observations. Dr. Maxey's original report on the "so-called spotted fever of Idaho" contains as vivid and accurate a description of the disease as has ever been published.

The history of the early studies on the disease in the Bitter Root Valley contains all the elements of rivalry and cooperation usually associated with a medical problem having political and economic overtones. The United States Public Health Service early entered into cooperation with the local authorities in Montana and Idaho, and this record serves as an excellent example of the type of federal intervention to be further emulated.

The hero of this story, of course, is Dr. Howard Taylor Ricketts. His genius has not been fully appreciated. Dr. Ricketts, of his own accord, went to the Bitter Root Valley because of sheer curiosity and the challenge of an unsolved medical problem. He accomplished much in a very short period. It is not generally recognized that, in his detailed, logical, often brilliant and original studies, he laid the groundwork and pattern for the conquest of all rickettsial diseases. One can only wonder how different would have been the course of medical research had the Montana Board of Examiners economized elsewhere and allowed Dr. Ricketts the funds originally appropriated for the continuation of his work.

The development of the programs for eradicating ticks and thus controlling the infection in human beings is a story of interdisciplinary cooperation involving many scientists, but the names of Spencer, Parker, and Cox stand out.

With the recognition of spotted fever in the eastern part of the United States, it becomes apparent that the organism existed in almost every state in the Union. What originally appeared to be a regional nuisance of the Rocky Mountain states has now been shown to be a worldwide problem, Rocky Mountain spotted fever itself being recognized in North and South America, and its kindred infections in Europe, South Africa, India, and Australia.

Understanding of the pathologic physiology of Rocky

Mountain spotted fever developed in prepared minds
as the disease moved eastward. Strange as it may seem,
there was a delay of more than twenty years before
Wolbach's detailed description of the pathologic anatomy
of the disease was applied to the understanding and
clinical management of its pathologic physiology. Harrell
deserves great credit for making this application.

The discovery of a cure for spotted fever represents
the final chapter of an epic. The urgent stimulus of a
major world conflict was required to effect this. With
the coming of World War II, the pharmaceutical industry
marshalled its resources and cooperated with the medical
profession and the federal government to solve medical
problems. The rise of American medicine to its present
preeminent position in the world is testimony to this joint
effort.

In some respects, the cure for Rocky Mountain spotted
fever came too soon. Even as radioisotopic tools became
available, making possible dynamic studies in physiology
and biochemistry, the antibiotics brought specific treatment and cure, and interest in spotted fever waned.

14.1 Unsolved Problems

From the evolutionary standpoint, the complex relationship between rickettsiae and ticks still remains to be
explained. In spite of the transovarial transmission of
R. rickettsii in the tick, the arthropod apparently suffers
no ill effects. How can this symbiotic relationship be
explained in terms of intracellular mechanisms? The
animal vectors also appear to be in symbiotic relationship
with the tick, and no clinical disease is evident. How does
one explain this in terms of biochemistry?

There must be a logical, biochemical, enzymatic

explanation for the unique intracellular, intranuclear localization of *R. rickettsii* in the endothelial cells and smooth muscles. Is this preference based on metabolic differences in specific tissues and organs? If so, what are these differences? Further pursuit of this subject may shed light on the peculiarities of the vascular structure that make it so susceptible to certain injuries, manifested clinically as cardiovascular diseases. Experimental Rocky Mountain spotted fever might be used as a tool in searching for such answers.

The recent reports on the effects of *R. rickettsii* on fibrinogen concentration merit detailed critical studies. The relationship between rickettsial infections and the clotting and lysing mechanisms of the blood also might be a fruitful unexplored field of research.

The changes in plasma volume and thiocyanate space observed in patients with spotted fever resemble those found in serum sickness. There is no doubt concerning the existence of a vascular lesion in the former condition; in the latter, an increase in permeability as a consequence of an intravascular antigen-antibody reaction has been suspected. The similarities noted in the two conditions might be the physiologic manifestations of biochemical lesions in the capillary endothelial cells or in the connective tissue. Since the immune or allergic reaction is a general response to exposure to any antigenic substance, further explorations of immunophysiology are indicated.

The concept that all clinical manifestations of Rocky Mountain spotted fever can be explained solely on the basis of direct endothelial damage resulting from the localization of the rickettsiae in the vascular system seems a rather mechanistic one. Whether it is correct or whether the immune mechanism contributes to the picture is still not known. What is the role of the rickettsial toxin? The soluble substance contains many characteristics of a heterophile antigen, including its apparent carbohydrate structure and thermostability. The role of the heterophile antigen in human disease has received scant attention. Electron microscopy has revealed the source of the soluble substance. Further utilization of this tool would furnish valuable information concerning the submicroscopic anatomy of the rickettsiae.

Many of the antibiotics inhibit the growth of rickettsiae. Cellular metabolism appears to be an interrelationship of many enzymatic processes in orderly sequence; just how and where in this chain do antibiotic agents exert their effects? Do they act primarily on the host cells or directly upon the rickettsiae? The tetracycline drugs, because of their fluorescence, can be detected in minute quantities; that they localize in bone and in nuclei and mitochondria is known. They appear to chelate magnesium. Are any of these observations related to the rickettsiostasis? Rickettsiae are visible by light microscopy. The dynamics of cellular metabolism can be traced with radioisotopes and radioautography. It appears that all of the tools essential for the synthesis of facts into a coherent explanation are now available for the prepared minds and hands that will pursue these intriguing problems further.

14.2 In Closing

So ends this factual story of the conquest of Rocky Mountain spotted fever. It is written now, before time obscures the memories of those who have worked with this disease, in the hope that its telling might bring pleasure and inspiration to all students of medicine, and pride tempered with humility to all Americans.

Rocky Mountain spotted fever should now be called *rickettsial spotted fever*, since it is no longer a regional curiosity but is of worldwide importance. It is fitting that the name of Howard Taylor Ricketts should be further honored in this way.

REFERENCES

1. Farb, P.: *Face of North America*. New York, Harper and Row, 1963.
2. Michie, H. C., Jr., and Parsons, H. H.: Rocky Mountain spotted (tick) fever. Report of an investigation in the Bitter Root Valley of Montana. *Med. Record*, 89:265, 1916.
3. Fricks, L. D.: Rocky Mountain spotted fever. A report of its investigation and of measures undertaken for its eradication during 1914. *Public Health Rep.*, 30:148, 1915.
4. Maxey, E. E.: Some observations on the so-called spotted fever of Idaho. *Med. Sentinel*, 7:433, 1899.
5. McCullough, G. T.: Spotted fever. *Med. Sentinel*, 10:225, 1902.
6. Anderson, J. F.: Spotted fever (tick fever) of the Rocky Mountains; a new disease. U. S. Public Health and Marine Hospital Service, *Hygienic Lab. Bull.*, 14, 1903.
7. Stiles, C. W.: A zoological investigation into the cause, transmission, and source of Rocky Mountain "spotted fever." U. S. Public Health and Marine Hospital Service, *Hygienic Lab. Bull.*, 20, 1905.
8. Price, E. G.: *Fighting Spotted Fever in the Rockies*. Helena, Naegele, 1948.
9. Wilson, L. B., and Chowning, W. M.: Studies in pyroplasmosis hominis ("spotted fever" or "tick fever" of the Rocky Mountains). *J. Infect. Dis.*, 1:31, 1904.
10. McCalla, L. P.: Direct transmission from man to man of the Rocky Mountain spotted (tick) fever. *Med. Sentinel*, 16:87, 1908.
11. Ricketts, H. T.: The study of "Rocky Mountain spotted

119

fever" (tick fever?) by means of animal inoculations. A preliminary communication. *J.A.M.A., 47*:33, 1906.

12. Ricketts, H. T.: The transmission of Rocky Mountain spotted fever by the bite of the wood-tick (Dermacentor occidentalis). *J.A.M.A., 47*:358, 1906.

13. Ricketts, H. T.: Further observations on Rocky Mountain spotted fever and Dermacentor occidentalis. *J.A.M.A., 47*:1067, 1906.

14. Ricketts, H. T.: Observations on the virus and means of transmission of Rocky Mountain spotted fever. *J. Infect. Dis., 4*:141, 1907.

15. Ricketts, H. T.: The role of the wood-tick (Dermacentor occidentalis) in Rocky Mountain spotted fever, and the susceptibility of local animals to this disease. A preliminary report. *J.A.M.A., 49*:24, 1907.

16. Ricketts, H. T., and Gomez, L.: Studies on immunity in Rocky Mountain spotted fever. *J. Infect. Dis., 5*:221, 1908.

17. Ricketts, H. T.: Some aspects of Rocky Mountain spotted fever as shown by recent investigations. *Med. Record, 76*:843, 1909.

18. Davis, B. F.: Unfinished experiments of Dr. Howard T. Ricketts on Rocky Mountain spotted fever. In Ricketts, H. T.: *Contributions to Medical Science.* Chicago, University of Chicago Press, 1911, p. 409-418.

19. Ricketts, H. T.: A micro-organism which apparently has a specific relationship to Rocky Mountain spotted fever. A preliminary report. *J.A.M.A., 52*:379, 1909.

20. Goodspeed, T. W.: Howard Taylor Ricketts. *The University Record, 8*:93, 1922.

21. Obituary. Howard Taylor Ricketts. *J.A.M.A., 54*:1640, 1910.

22. Hektoen, L.: Howard Taylor Ricketts, 1871-1910. *Quart. Bull. Northw. Univ. Med. Sch., 19*:2, 1945.

23. Ricketts, H. T.: *Contributions to Medical Science.* Chicago, University of Chicago Press, 1911.

24. Cutler, I. S.: Howard Taylor Ricketts, 1871-1910. *Quart. Bull. Northw. Univ. Med. Sch.*, *19*:1, 1945.
25. Birdseye, C.: Some common mammals of Western Montana in relation to agriculture and spotted fever. *U. S. Dept. Agric. Farmers Bull.*, *484*:1, 1912.
26. King, W. W.: Experimental transmission of Rocky Mountain spotted fever by means of the tick. Preliminary note. *Public Health Rep.*, *21*:863, 1906.
27. McClintic, T. B.: Investigations of and tick eradication in Rocky Mountain spotted fever. *Public Health Rep.*, *27*:732, 1912.
28. Cooley, R. A.: The spotted fever tick (Dermacentor venustus Banks) and its control in the Bitter Root Valley, Montana. A review. *J. Economic Entomol.*, *8*:47, 1915.
29. Fricks, L. D.: Rocky Mountain spotted (or tick) fever. Sheep grazing as a possible means of controlling the wood tick (Dermacentor andersoni) in the Bitter Root Valley. *Public Health Rep.*, *28*:1647, 1913.
30. Parker, R. R.: Some results of two years' investigations of the Rocky Mountain spotted fever tick in eastern Montana. *J. Economic Entomol.*, *11*:189, 1918.
31. LeCount, E. R.: A contribution to the pathological anatomy of Rocky Mountain spotted fever. *J. Infect. Dis.*, *8*:421, 1911.
32. Wolbach, S. B.: Studies on Rocky Mountain spotted fever. *J. Med. Res.*, *41*:1, 1919.
33. Wolbach, S. B.: The etiology of Rocky Mountain spotted fever. A preliminary report. *J. Med. Res.*, *34*:121, 1916.
34. Parker, R. R.: The present status of the control of Dermacentor venustus Banks in the Bitter Root Valley, Montana, and new data concerning the habits of the tick. *J. Economic Entomol.*, *13*:31, 1920.
35. Parker, R. R.: Transmission of Rocky Mountain spotted fever by the rabbit tick Haemaphysalis leporis palus-

tris Packard. *Amer. J. Trop. Med.*, 3:39, 1923.

36. Spencer, R. R., and Parker, R. R.: Rocky Mountain spotted fever: Infectivity of fasting and recently fed ticks. *Public Health Rep.*, 38:333, 1923.

37. Spencer, R. R., and Parker, R. R.: Rocky Mountain spotted fever: Vaccination of monkeys and man. *Public Health Rep.*, 40:2159, 1925.

38. Parker, R. R., and Spencer, R. R.: Studies on Rocky Mountain spotted fever. Results of four years' human vaccination. U. S. Public Health Service, *Hygienic Lab. Bull.*, 154:72, 1930.

39. Parker, R. R.: Rocky Mountain spotted fever. Results of ten years' prophylactic vaccination. *J. Infect. Dis.*, 57:78, 1935.

40. Parker, R. R.: Rocky Mountain spotted fever. Results of fifteen years' prophylactic vaccination. *Amer. J. Trop. Med.*, 21:369, 1941.

41. Parker, R. R., and Steinhaus, E. A.: Rocky Mountain spotted fever: Duration of potency of tick-tissue vaccine. *Pub. Health Rep.*, 58:230, 1943.

42. Noguchi, H.: Prophylactic inoculation against Rocky Mountain spotted fever. Special Bull. No. 26, Montana State Board of Health, Helena, p. 44-47, 1923.

43. Noguchi, H.: Experimental prophylactic inoculation against Rocky Mountain spotted fever. *Northw. Med.*, 22:301, 1923.

44. Pierce, C. M., and Vanderkamp, H.: Rocky Mountain spotted fever. Report of two cases in Western Nebraska. *Nebraska Med. J.*, 16:69, 1931.

45. Maver, M. B.: Transmission of spotted fever by the tick in nature. *J. Infect. Dis.*, 8:327, 1911.

46. Dyer, R. E.: Rumreich, A. S., and Badger, L. F.: The typhus-Rocky Mountain spotted fever group in the United States, *J.A.M.A.*, 97:589, 1931.

47. Brigham, G. D., and Watt, J.: Highly virulent strains of Rocky Mountain spotted fever virus isolated from

ticks (D. variabilis) in Georgia. *Public Health Rep.*, 55:2125, 1940.

48. Topping, N. H., and Dyer, R. E.: A highly virulent strain of Rocky Mountain spotted fever virus isolated in the Eastern United States. *Public Health Rep.*, 55:728, 1940.

49. Lillie, R. D.: Pathology of the Eastern type of Rocky Mountain spotted fever. *Public Health Rep.*, 46:2840, 1931.

50. Harris, P. N.: Histological study of a case of the Eastern type of Rocky Mountain spotted fever. *Amer. J. Path.*, 9:91, 1933.

51. Dyer, R. E., Badger, L. F., and Rumreich, A.: Rocky Mountain spotted fever (Eastern type). Transmission by the American dog tick (Dermacentor variabilis). *Public Health Rep.*, 46:1403, 1931.

52. Badger, L. F.: Rocky Mountain spotted fever (Eastern type). Virus recovered from the dog tick Dermacentor variabilis found in nature. *Public Health Rep.*, 47:2365, 1932.

53. Badger, L. F.: Rocky Mountain spotted fever: Susceptibility of the dog and sheep to the virus. *Public Health Rep.*, 48:791, 1933.

54. Parker, R. R., Philip, C. B., and Jellison, W. L.: Rocky Mountain spotted fever. Potentialities of tick transmission in relation to geographical occurrence in the United States. *Amer. J. Trop. Med.*, 13:341, 1933.

55. Cumming, J. G.: Rocky Mountain spotted fever invades the East. *Southern Med. J.*, 27:783, 1934.

56. Kemp, H. A., and Grigsby, C. M.: The occurrence and identification of an infection of the Rocky Mountain spotted fever type in Texas. *Texas J. Med.*, 27:395, 1931.

57. Piza, J., Salles-Gomes, F., Salles-Gomes, L., Meyer, J., Fleury, J. P., Castro, O., Rodrigues, C., and Lima,

H. R.: Le typhus exanthématique à San Paulo, *C. R. Soc. Biol. (Par.)*, *106*:1020, 1931.

58. Patino, L., Afanador, A., and Paul, J. H.: A spotted fever in Tobia, Columbia. Preliminary report. *Amer. J. Trop. Med.*, *17*:639, 1937.

59. Hearle, E.: The ticks of British Columbia. *Sci. Agric.*, *18*:341, 1938.

60. Bustamante, M. E., and Varela, G.: Una nueva rickettsiosis en Mexico. *Rev. Inst. Salubr. Enferm. Trop.*, *4*:189, 1943.

61. De Rodaniche, E. C., and Rodaniche, A.: Spotted fever in Panama; isolation of the etiologic agent from a fatal case. *Amer. J. Trop. Med.*, *30*:511, 1950.

62. Wolbach, S. B., Pinkerton, H., and Schlesinger, M. J.: The cultivation of the organism of Rocky Mountain spotted fever and typhus in tissue cultures. *Proc. Soc. Exp. Biol. Med.*, *20*:270, 1922.

63. Wolbach, S. B., and Schlesinger, M. J.: The cultivation of the micro-organisms of Rocky Mountain spotted fever (Dermacentroxenus rickettsi) and of typhus (Rickettsia prowazeki) in tissue plasma cultures. *J. Med. Res.*, *44*:231, 1923.

64. Rous, P., and Murphy, J. B.: Tumor implantations in the developing embryo; experiments with a transmissible sarcoma of the fowl. *J.A.M.A.*, *57*:741, 1911.

65. Woodruff, A. M., and Goodpasture, E. W.: The susceptibility of the chorio-allantoic membrane of chick embryos to infection with the fowl-pox virus. *Amer. J. Path.*, *7*:209, 1931.

66. Bengtson, I. A., and Dyer, R. E.: Cultivation of the virus of Rocky Mountain spotted fever in the developing chick embryo. *Public Health Rep.*, *50*:1489, 1935.

67. Lillie, R. D.: Histologic reaction to the virus of Rocky Mountain spotted fever in chick embryos. *Public Health Rep.*, *50*:1498, 1935.

68. Cox, H. R.: Use of yolk sac of developing chick embryo

as medium for growing rickettsiae of Rocky Mountain spotted fever and typhus groups. *Public Health Rep.*, 53:2241, 1938.

69. Cox, H. R.: Cultivation of rickettsiae of the Rocky Mountain spotted fever, typhus and Q fever groups in the embryonic tissues of developing chicks. *Science, 94:* 339, 1941.

70. Greiff, D., Pinkerton, H., and Moragues, V.: Effect of enzyme inhibitors and activators on the multiplication of typhus rickettsiae. *J. Exp. Med., 80:*561, 1944.

71. Cox, H. R.: Growth of viruses and rickettsiae in the developing chick embryo. *Ann. N. Y. Acad. Sci., 55:*236, 1952.

72. Pinkerton, H.: The study of typhus and Rocky Mountain spotted fever by the tissue culture method. *Arch. F. Exp. Zellforsch., 15:*425, 1934.

73. Pinkerton, H., and Hass, G. M.: Spotted fever. 1. Intranuclear rickettsiae in spotted fever studied in tissue culture. *J. Exp. Med., 56:*151, 1932.

74. Smadel, J. E.: Complement-fixation and agglutination reactions in rickettsial diseases. In Moulton, F. R.: *Rickettsial Diseases of Man.* Washington, American Association for the Advancement of Science, 1948, p. 190-197.

75. Pinkerton, H.: The classification of rickettsiae and rickettsial diseases. In Moulton, F. R.: *Rickettsial Diseases of Man.* Washington, American Association for the Advancement of Science, 1948, p. 64-75.

76. Wertman, K.: The Weil-Felix reaction. In Moulton, F. R.: *The Rickettsial Diseases of Man.* Washington, American Association for the Advancement of Science, 1948, p. 184-189.

77. Felix, A.: Die Serodiagnostik des Fleckfiebers. *Wien. Klin. Wschr., 29:*873, 1916.

78. Kelly, F. L.: Weil-Felix reaction in Rocky Mountain spotted fever. *J. Infect. Dis., 32:*223, 1923.

79. Kerlee, A. L., and Spencer, R. R.: Rocky Mountain spotted fever; a preliminary report on the Weil-Felix reaction. *Public Health Rep.*, *44*:179, 1929.
80. Munter, H.: Über die Weil-Felixsche Reaktion beim experimentellen Felsen-gebirgsfieber. *Z. Hyg. Infektionskr.*, *109*:124, 1928.
81. Spencer, R. R., and Maxcy, K. F.: The Weil-Felix reaction in endemic typhus fever and in Rocky Mountain spotted fever. *Public Health Rep.*, *45*:440, 1930.
82. Davis, G. E., and Parker, R. R.: Observations on the agglutination of Proteus X organisms in Rocky Mountain spotted fever. *Public Health Rep.*, *47*:1511, 1932.
83. Davis, G. E., Parker, R. R., and Walker, M. E.: Further observations on the agglutination of Proteus X strains in Rocky Mountain spotted fever. *Public Health Rep.*, *49*:298, 1934.
84. Plotz, H.: The interpretation of the Weil-Felix agglutination test in Rocky Mountain spotted fever. *J. Lab. Clin. Med.*, *31*:982, 1946.
85. Parker, R. R.: Rocky Mountain spotted fever. *J.A.M.A.*, *110*:1185-1273, 1938.
86. Bengtson, I. A.: Complement fixation in endemic typhus fever. *Public Health Rep.*, *56*:649, 1941.
87. Craigie, J.: Application and control of ethyl-ether-water interface effects to the separation of rickettsiae from yolk sac suspensions. *Canad. J. Res. 23*:104, 1945.
88. Plotz, H.: Complement fixation in rickettsial diseases. *Science, 97*:20, 1943.
89. Davis, B. F., and Petersen, W. F.: Complement deviation in Rocky Mountain spotted fever. *J. Infect. Dis.*, *8*:330, 1911.
90. Plotz, H., and Wertman, K.: The use of the complement fixation test in Rocky Mountain spotted fever. *Science, 95*:441, 1942.
91. Plotz, H., Wertman, K., and Reagan, R. L.: Laboratory aids in diagnosis of Rocky Mountain spotted fever.

Bull. U. S. Army Med. Dept., 79:40, 1944.

92. Plotz, H., Wertman, K., and Bennett, B. L.: Identification of rickettsial agents isolated in guinea pigs by means of specific complement fixation. *Proc. Soc. Exp. Biol. Med.,* 61:76, 1946.

93. Bengtson, I. A.: Applications of the complement fixation test in the study of rickettsial diseases. *Amer. J. Public Health,* 35:701, 1945.

94. Fitzpatrick, F., and Hampil, B.: Immunological reactions in rickettsial diseases with special reference to the time of appearance of antibodies. *Amer. J. Public Health,* 31:1301, 1941.

95. Castaneda, M. R.: The antigenic relationship between Proteus X-19 and typhus rickettsia. *J. Exp. Med.,* 60: 119, 1943.

96. Cohen, S. S., and Chargaff, E.: Studies on the composition of Rickettsia prowazeki. *J. Biol. Chem.,* 154:691, 1944.

97. Topping, N. H., and Shear, M. J.: Studies of antigens in infected yolk sacs. *Nat. Inst. Health Bull.,* 183:13, 1945.

98. Plotz, H.: The soluble substances of the rickettsiae. In Moulton, F. R.: *Rickettsial Diseases of Man.* Washington, American Association for the Advancement of Science, 1948, p. 198-202.

99. Shepard, C. C., and Wyckoff, R. W. G.: The nature of the soluble antigen from typhus rickettsiae. *Public Health Rep.,* 61:761, 1946.

100. Bell, E. J., and Pickens, E. G.: A toxic substance associated with the rickettsias of the spotted fever group. *J. Immun.,* 70:461, 1953.

101. Chang, R. S., Murray, E. S., and Snyder, J. C.: Erythrocyte-sensitizing substances from rickettsiae of the Rocky Mountain spotted fever group. *J. Immun.,* 73:8, 1954.

102. Mel'nikov, L. A.: The serological diagnosis of rickettsi-

oses of the typhus and tick-borne spotted fever group by the haemagglutination method. II. The specificity of the reaction. *Problems of Virology,* 4:10, 1959.

103. Coons, A. H., Snyder, J. C., Cheever, F. S., and Murray, E. S.: Localization of antigen in tissue cells. IV. Antigens of rickettsiae and mumps virus. *J. Exp. Med., 91*:31, 1950.

104. Burgdorfer, W., and Lackman, D.: Identification of Rickettsia rickettsii in the wood tick, Dermacentor andersoni, by means of fluorescent antibody. *J. Infect. Dis., 107*:241, 1960.

105. Shepard, C. C., and Goldwasser, R. A.: Fluorescent antibody staining as a means of detecting Rocky Mountain spotted fever infection in individual ticks. *Amer. J. Hyg., 72*:120, 1960.

106. Fleck, L.: Specific antigenic substances in the urine of typhus patients. *Texas Rep. Biol. Med.,* 5:168, 1947.

107. Drobyshevskaya, A. I., and Smorodintzeff, A. A.: Early diagnosis of typhus fever through detection of specific antigen by complement-fixation test. *J. Epid. Microbiol. (Moscow),* No. 1, 1942.

108. Smorodintzeff, A. A., and Fradkina, R. V.: Slide agglutination test for rapid diagnosis of pre-eruptive typhus fever. *Proc. Soc. Exp. Biol. Med., 56*:93, 1944.

109. Aikawa, J. K., and Harrell, G. T.: Unpublished data.

110. Harrell, G. T., Venning, W., and Wolff, W. A.: The treatment of Rocky Mountain spotted fever with particular reference to intravenous fluids. A new approach to basic supportive therapy. *J.A.M.A., 126*:929, 1944.

111. Topping, N. H.: Rocky Mountain spotted fever. *Med. Clin. N. Amer., 27*:722, 1943.

112. Martin, D. W., Rocky Mountain spotted fever in children. *J. Pediat., 16*:468, 1940.

113. Harrell, G. T., Wolff, W. A., and Venning, W.: A new approach to basic supportive therapy in Rocky Mountain spotted fever. *Southern Med. J.,* 38:367, 1945.

114. Harrell, G. T., and Aikawa, J. K.: Pathogenesis of circulatory failure in Rocky Mountain spotted fever. *Arch. Intern. Med.*, 83:331, 1949.
115. Harrell, G. T., Wolff, W. A., Venning, W. L., and Reinhard, J. B.: The prevention and control of disturbances of protein metabolism in Rocky Mountain spotted fever. *Southern Med. J.*, 39:551, 1946.
116. Harrell, G. T., Aikawa, J. K., and Kelsey, W. M.: Rocky Mountain spotted fever. *Amer. Practit.*, 1:425, 1947.
117. Aikawa, J. K., and Harrell, G. T.: The immunophysiology of serum sickness. Alterations in the blood volume and thiocyanate space in relation to the development of humoral antibodies in the rabbit. *J. Clin. Invest.*, 30:360, 1951.
118. Aikawa, J. K., and Harrell, G. T.: Isotopic studies of fluid and electrolyte changes in domestic rabbits with Rocky Mountain spotted fever. *J. Infect. Dis.*, 93:222, 1953.
119. Aikawa, J. K., and Harrell, G. T.: Changes in the tissue radiosodium space associated with experimental Rocky Mountain spotted fever in guinea pigs. *J. Infect. Dis.*, 93:263, 1953.
120. Aikawa, J. K., and Rhoades, E. L.: Immunophysiology. Increase in radiosodium space of adrenal glands in rabbits sensitized with human plasma. *Proc. Soc. Exp. Biol. Med.*, 79:233, 1952.
121. Aquilina, J. T., Rosenberg, F., and Wuertz, R. L.: Nodal tachycardia in a case of Rocky Mountain spotted fever. *Amer. Heart J.*, 43:755, 1952.
122. Phillips, C. W., Jr., Kimbrough, G. T., Weaver, J. A., and Tucker, A. L.: Rocky Mountain spotted fever with thrombocytopenia. *Southern Med. J.*, 53:867, 1960.
123. Mengel, C. E., and Trygstad, C.: Thrombocytopenia in Rocky Mountain spotted fever. *J.A.M.A.*, 183:886, 1963.
124. Trigg, J. W., Jr.: Hypofibrinogenemia in Rocky Moun-

tain spotted fever. Report of a case. *New Engl. J. Med.*, *270*:1042, 1964.

125. Thomas, M. H., and Berlin, L.: Neurologic sequelae of Rocky Mountain spotted fever. *Arch. Neurol. Psychiat.*, *60*:574, 1948.

126. Rosenblum, M. J., Masland, R. L., and Harrell, G. T.: Residual effects of rickettsial disease on the central nervous system. Results of neurologic examinations and electroencephalograms following Rocky Mountain spotted fever. *Arch. Intern. Med.*, *90*:444, 1952.

127. Harrell, G. T.: Rickettsial involvement of the nervous system. *Med. Clin. N. Amer.*, *37*:395, 1953.

128. Baker, G. E.: Rocky Mountain spotted fever. *Med. Clin. N. Amer.*, *35*:907, 1951.

129. McCroan, J. E., Ramsey, R. L., Murphy, W. J., and Dick, L. S.: The status of Rocky Mountain spotted fever in the Southeastern United States. *Public Health Rep.*, *70*:319, 1955.

130. Topping, N. H.: Rocky Mountain spotted fever. Treatment of infected laboratory animals with immune rabbit serum. *Public Health Rep.*, *55*:41, 1940.

131. Topping, N. H.: Rocky Mountain spotted fever. Further experience in the therapeutic use of immune rabbit serum. *Public Health Rep.*, *58*:757, 1943.

132. Topping, N. H.: Experimental Rocky Mountain spotted fever and endemic typhus treated with Prontosil or sulfapyridine. *Public Health Rep.*, *54*:1143, 1939.

133. Fitzpatrick, F. K.: Penicillin in experimental spotted fever. *Science*, *102*:96, 1945.

134. Snyder, J. C., Maier, J., and Anderson, C. R.: Report to the Division of Medical Sciences, National Research Council, Dec. 26, 1942.

135. Greiff, D., Pinkerton, H., and Moragues, V.: Effect of enzyme inhibitors and activators on the multiplication of typhus rickettsiae. I. Penicillin, para-aminobenzoic

acid, sodium fluoride, and vitamins of the B group. *J. Exp. Med., 80*:561, 1944.

136. Yeomans, A., Snyder, J. C., Murray, E. S., Zarafonetis, C. J. D., and Ecke, R. S.: The therapeutic effect of para-aminobenzoic acid in louse-borne typhus fever. *J.A.M.A., 126*:349, 1944.

137. Anigstein, L., and Bader, M. N.: Para-aminobenzoic acid —its effectiveness in spotted fever in guinea pigs. *Science, 101*:591, 1945.

138. Hamilton, H. L.: Effect of p-aminobenzoic acid on growth of rickettsiae and elementary bodies, with observations on mode of action. *Proc. Soc. Exp. Biol. Med., 59*:220, 1945.

139. Rose, H. M., Duane, R. B., and Fischel, E. E.: The treatment of spotted fever with para-aminobenzoic acid. *J.A.M.A., 129*:1160, 1945.

140. Maroney, J. W., Davis, H. C., and Scott, E. G.: Rocky Mountain spotted fever: A case treated with p-aminobenzoic acid. *Delaware Med. J., 18*:104, 1946.

141. Flinn, L. B., Howard, J. W., Todd, C. W., and Scott, E. G.: Para-aminobenzoic acid treatment of Rocky Mountain spotted fever. *J.A.M.A., 132*:911, 1946.

142. Ravenel, S. F.: Para-aminobenzoic acid therapy of Rocky Mountain spotted fever. *J.A.M.A., 133*:989, 1947.

143. Woodward, T. E., and Raby, W. T.: Further concepts in the treatment of Rocky Mountain spotted fever with para-aminobenzoic acid. *Southern Med. J., 41*: 997, 1948.

144. Peterson, O. L.: Therapeutic effects of Forbisen and toluidine blue on experimental typhus. *Proc. Soc. Exp. Biol. Med., 55*:155, 1944.

145. Greiff, D., and Pinkerton, H.: Effect of enzyme inhibitors and activators on the multiplication of typhus rickettsiae. III. Correlation of effects of PABA and KCN with oxygen consumption in embryonate eggs. *J. Exp. Med., 87*:175, 1948.

146. Greiff, D.: Biology of the rickettsiae. In Moulton, F. R.: *Rickettsial Diseases of Man.* Washington, American Association for the Advancement of Science 1948, p. 51-63.

147. Duggar, B. M. Aureomycin: A product of the continuing search for new antibiotics. *Ann. N. Y. Acad. Sci., 51:* 177, 1948.

148. Wong, S. C., and Cox, H. R.: Action of Aureomycin against experimental rickettsial and viral infections. *Ann. N. Y. Acad. Sci., 51:*290, 1948.

149. Ross, S., Schoenbach, E. B., Burke, F. G., Bryer, M. S., Rice, E. C., and Washington, J. A.: Aureomycin therapy of Rocky Mountain spotted fever. *J.A.M.A., 138:* 1213, 1948.

150. Ehrlich, J., Bartz, Q R., Smith, R. M., Joslyn, D. A., and Burkholder, P. R.: Chloromycetin, a new antibiotic from a soil actinomycete. *Science, 106:*417, 1947.

151. Smith, R. M., Joslyn, D. A., Gruhzit, O. M., McLean, W. I., Jr., Penner, M. A., and Ehrlich, J.: Chloromycetin: biologic studies. *J. Bact. 55:*425, 1948.

152. Smadel, J. E., and Jackson, E. B.: Chloromycetin, an antibiotic with chemotherapeutic activity in experimental rickettsial and viral infections. *Science, 106:* 418, 1947.

153. Pincoffs, M. C., Guy, E. G., Lister, L. M., Woodward, T. E., and Smadel, J. E.: The treatment of Rocky Mountain spotted fever with Chloromycetin. *Ann. Intern. Med., 29:*656, 1948.

154. Smadel, J. E.: The changing status of the rickettsioses. *Trans. Amer. Clin. Climat. Ass., 61:*152, 1949.

155. Parker, R. T., Menon, P. G., Merideth, A. M., Snyder, M. J., and Woodward, T. E.: Persistence of Rickettsia rickettsii in a patient recovered from Rocky Mountain spotted fever. *J. Immun., 73:*383, 1954.

156. Finlay, A. C., Hobby, G. L., P'an, S. Y., Regna, P. P.,

Routien, J. B., Seeley, D. B., Shull, G. M., Sobin, B. A., Solomons, I. A., Vinson, J. W., and Kane, J. H.: Terramycin, a new antibiotic. *Science,* 111:85, 1950.

157. Bauer, R. E., Parker, R. T., Hall, H. E., Benson, J. F., Joslin, B. S., Hightower, J. A., Snyder, M. J., Venable, S. J., and Woodward, T. E.: Clinical and experimental observations with Terramycin in certain rickettsial and bacterial infections. *Ann. N. Y. Acad. Sci.,* 53:395, 1950.

158. Brody, T. M.: The uncoupling of oxidative phosphorylation as a mechanism of drug action. *Pharmacol. Rev.,* 7:335, 1955.

159. Eisenhardt, R. H., and Rosenthal, O.: 2,4-Dinitrophenol: Lack of interaction with high-energy intermediates of oxidative phosphorylation. *Science,* 143:476, 1964.

160. Buyske, D. A., Eisner, H. J., and Kelly, R. G.: Concentration and persistence of tetracycline and chlortetracycline in bone. *J. Pharmacol. Exp. Ther.,* 130:150, 1960.

161. du Buy, H. G., and Showacre, J. L.: Selective localization of tetracycline in mitochondria of living cells. *Science,* 133:196, 1961.

162. Smith, M. H.: Rocky Mountain spotted fever treated with adrenal secretion. *Med. Record,* 88:568, 1915.

163. Aikawa, J. K., and Harrell, G. T.: Effect of cortisone acetate on experimental Rocky Mountain spotted fever in the guinea pig. *Proc. Soc. Exp. Biol. Med.,* 82:698, 1953.

164. Kass, E. H., Ingbar, S. H., and Finland, M.: Effects of adrenocorticotropic hormone in pneumonia: Clinical, bacteriological and serological studies. *Ann. Intern. Med.,* 33:1081, 1950.

165. Arney, W. C.: Cortisone and Aureomycin in the treatment of a case of Rocky Mountain spotted fever. *N. Carolina Med. J.,* 13:29, 1952.

166. Workman, J. B., Hightower, J. A., Borges, F. J., Furman,

J. E., and Parker, R. T.: Cortisone as an adjunct to chloramphenicol in the treatment of Rocky Mountain spotted fever. *New Engl. J. Med.*, *246*:962, 1952.

167. McCroan, J. E., Ramsey, R. L., Murphy, W. J., and Dick, L. S.: The status of Rocky Mountain spotted fever in the Southeastern United States. *Public Health Rep.*, 70:319, 1955.

168. Flinn, L. B.: A review of Rocky Mountain spotted fever in Delaware. *Delaware Med. J.*, 29:41, 1957.

Index

135